BE
YOUR
SELF
AND
HAPPIER

BE YOUR SELF

AND

HAPPIER

THE A–Z OF WELLBEING

WILL YOUNG

**EBURY
SPOTLIGHT**

Introduction

Be Yourself and Happier is an idea I have been working on for six years now.

In 2011, I had a breakdown. When I realised I was actually having one – something I had heard whispers about but never truly observed – I felt almost relieved, and special.

I am in the middle of a full-on breakdown, I would think to myself. *I am actually experiencing it RIGHT NOW!*

What a thing to behold. People talk about life after a breakdown but not often when they are in the middle of one. Looking back, I wish I had crowed about it even more. I mean, I did inform quite a varied group of people – from taxi drivers to the local barista.

'A soya latte, please, and just to make you aware, Stephen … I'm currently in the midst of my very own mental breakdown,' I would utter with a little secretive smile as if I was letting him into a very special club of my own.

One of my favourite comments from my therapist at that time was:

'You think your dog is judging you? Are you fucking insane?'

There were other things said which I can't repeat ...

I jest, and yet of course it was absolutely terrifying and horrific. I would crawl around the square where I used to live, walking my new Border terrier, Esme, and would literally be bent over double with agoraphobia. Poor Esme.

I went about the process of completely disassembling everything I thought was correct in my world – how I had formed my identity; what I relied on for self-esteem; what I thought made me worthwhile; how I behaved; how I communicated – finding who I truly was. I read a lot of books and did a lot of therapy and, during this time, my mind started to wish that all the information I needed was all in one place. And so here it is!

My title is perhaps a bit forward; too emboldened or even arrogant. I do truly believe, however, that these snippets of wisdom and explanations of symptoms, disorders and behaviours might just help you – the reader – resonate with a few and see some things inside yourself and others that will perhaps explain certain thought patterns – and even allow you to find some relief. Everything I have learnt over the last ten years I have tried to condense into this small book. Stuff that I believe is truly invaluable to leading an authentic and appropriate adult life. Life isn't easy and so often I was confused as to why I found it so hard – beyond the usual day-to-day challenges. I have accrued all this knowledge I have gained and look to pass it on to you, dear reader, with love and honesty.

When I started therapy fifteen years ago, there were many things I didn't understand, and I often found books over-intellectualised and obviously written more for other academics and professionals than people like me. And then there were other books that over-simplified the problem. For example: mindfulness. It is without doubt a wonderful tool, yet when the body is overrun with traumatic energy and a part of the brain is firing on all cylinders, telling you that you're about to die, it is very difficult to be mindful of the petals on a fucking flower. Words like 'co-dependency' and 'boundaries' – what do they actually mean? What is a 'trigger'? I wanted to explore these things and show the meanings of and potential value in all of them, and also perhaps open up the different worlds of types of therapies that are on offer, therapies that go beyond just the mind and look to calm the body.

There is nothing in this little guidebook that I have not tried or dived into myself. I am, if you like, my very own litmus test. Everything I share, I share from a place of honest experience and feelings – from body image to breathing, shamans to somatic therapy! There is SO much out there to explore, and my motto has always been that I only get one life so I'm going to try my damndest to be as content and peaceful as I can be.

I appreciate that not all the techniques discussed in the book will be accessible or applicable to everyone, but I hope you will find something that resonates or is useful.

I also want to state at this point that everyone will experience the issues I discuss differently based on their own situation, so I have stuck to my personal experiences in the hope that you can take that and apply it to your own situation, if helpful.

No one really knows why some people find their way more than others. But I believe that for those of us who do suffer from bouts of poor mental health, our stories are much more than what has happened to us. Our struggles do not define us, yet – in time and with practice – we can come to see them as strengths, as a part of our nature. What I do know for sure is that we are all made of beautiful, wonderful stuff. We are all our very own walking miracle. In this book I have come across things that have reminded me of that, and I believe everyone can move closer to a place of sensing their own magical make-up and look to be in touch with their own inner beauty and wonder. We are born pure and then stuff can get put on us: our nervous system moulds, then our belief system; attachment causes us to act a certain way and hold on to deep beliefs that we must unravel, understand, accept and nurture, before we finally allow ourselves to rise with our vulnerabilities – not despite them.

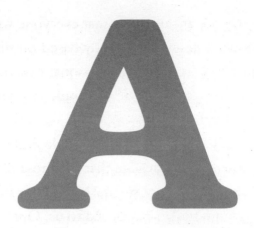

Activation

I came to the concept of activation when I started trauma therapy and really looked at how my nervous system was responding. Put simply, if I was activated I was normally in some level of a fight-or-flight or a freeze-or-faint response. It is a heightened response to stuff we feel in our body. Often it will be in response to uncomfortable feelings, but the annoying thing for me was that this activation was just as uncomfortable! If I was in fight-or-flight mode, I would normally disassociate and potentially get brain fog, and if I was in a freeze-or-faint response I would go into depression and again have brain fog.

Activation is like a fizz around the body. I say it's like I'm freewheeling on a bike – where I'm pedalling and the chain has come off the wheel – so a lot of energy is being created, yet I'm going nowhere. To think of it as simply activation in my body can remove any notion of being tied to a certain narrative like 'I don't have anyone who likes me', 'I'm just useless and a piece of shit' or 'my house is horrible'; whatever the story is, we can often bypass that and go straight to the source of activation. This is why when people come to me in a state of anxiety, I will often immediately suggest treating the body as well as the mind, or even before the mind. The activation is controlling their life so they need help to bring that down, perhaps through massage, cranial osteopathy, acupuncture or sound therapy. Once the body is calm we often find that the problems we felt we had aren't really problems at all; our brain was just looking for a reason to explain the high levels of cortisol.

Someone told me years ago that I was not my story and I laughed in his face. How could I not be my story? My story is my story. It got me realising, though, that it is just a narrative, it doesn't have to be my life. Looking at activation in my body and how energy swells up and what allows it to dissipate has started me on my path of noticing when I'm activated, trying to disengage with the thoughts associated with it, and quelling the activation so that I can carry on with my day.

When we visit a shaman, they are not that interested in the story. In fact, shamans, through many different methods, look at our energy, our activation, and then move the energy around to find calm, peace and tranquillity, along with the ability to rest in our own power. It's an astonishing thing and, really, it is science. By learning to calm our activation, we learn self-mastery, and this is where we want to be in life. We want to be the captain of our ship and have the ability to ride the inevitable storms that come our way.

Adult

One of my favourite words. My old therapist Lois Evans, the most fantastic Jewish New Yorker – who I often asked, 'Lois, have I paid for those Tiffany earrings?' – said her aim was to get her clients to a place of becoming a functional adult; a person who acts with containment, emotional awareness and appropriateness. It is good to ask oneself, 'Am I actually acting like an adult right now?' and 'Am I throwing a childish strop, screaming obscenities at people?' or even just 'Am I eating properly?'

I ran through the park a while ago and a man in his fifties threw his rubbish on the ground right by a bin. I told him to put it in the bin. He shouted, 'Fuck off,' at me and my reply was to ask how old he was. While I felt rather smug with my put-down and safe because I was on the move, it is also a basic question to someone: 'Are you REALLY going to act like this??'

Often our upbringing is guided by adult children, i.e. parents, who aren't fully formed functional adults, so we are frequently denied the opportunity to actually learn, or be shown an example of, what it is to be a functional adult in this world. It is never too late, however …

Adult Children

Here is a little test and include yourself in it ... take a look around you and in the mirror and ask yourself how many adult children you see and experience on a daily basis. They could be your neighbour, your partner, your kids, your friends, your work colleagues ... the list is endless.

An adult child is basically in a state of arrested development. This can be for many reasons, but essentially, if we haven't resolved younger parts of ourselves – like the four-year-old who got shamed constantly, or the thirteen-year-old who got bullied – we grow up into a child in an adult body. How can we identify this in ourselves and others? Essentially by our actions. The partner that throws a tantrum or the neighbour who is in a state of panic if you decide to put up a satellite dish. Look at children's behaviour and see if you identify it in any adults. You will.

Adult children can be vulnerable and uncontained, and they can also act out and be extremely dangerous because they have a lot more at their disposal than perhaps a kid of six who is throwing a tantrum does. They can be extremely toxic and this often leads to narcissism and even psychopathic tendencies. Donald Trump is, in my opinion, the most obvious adult child.

How do we deal with them? We need to set clear boundaries as we would with a kid. We set boundaries and we let them know what the consequences of their actions will be. So many people have terrified, scared, sad and angry children inside them, and by not recognising this, they can lash out. Check in with yourself: are you an adult child? Are you happy or acting out, and what needs to be done to maintain your inner child's peace and tranquillity?

Advice

'Advice': a seemingly harmful word. In fact, quite the opposite. I shall quote the *Oxford English Dictionary*: 'guidance or recommendations offered with regard to prudent action'.

What I noticed after becoming a famous pop singer is that people wanted to give their advice a LOT of the time: in the butcher's, on the bus ... even at a funeral. It started with the phrase 'The thing is, Will, you SHOULD ...' (That word, which we shall dissect later.)

Here are some suggestions about advice if you are open to them, dear reader:

1 Ask people if they are open to your advice, and equally, if someone starts splurging their opinion at you and you haven't asked for it, tell them that you do not want to hear their opinion, thank you very much. An example from my life is that, after a concert, people would often come storming into my dressing room with immediate words of wisdom. I was too vulnerable at that stage and not asking for it, so slowly I learnt to set boundaries and say no, I was tired and oversensitive so was not open to hearing feedback. It is not for ANYONE to force their opinion or advice on another EVER, even if the intention is coming from the kindest of places.

2 Be careful who you ask for advice. I have a rule …
I have five people (max) who I ask for advice on
stuff. In regards to emotional awareness, that probably
goes down to three, for cooking tips one (the mother,
of course). Choose who you ask very selectively. Are
you asking people who will really understand? Are they
people who will really listen to you? Will they just tell you
what you want to hear or, conversely, will they just think
about themselves? Don't ask too many people either; this
can cloud the water, especially if you find making decisions hard. You can voice to people stuff that you feel
needs to be got out there; however, do not ask EVERY
person for their input.

3 Finally, often we know the answer within us. If we
really check in with ourselves, what does our gut tell
us? People call the gut the second brain (for more on
this, see 'Instinct' on page 115). I like to call it the first.
It shows us the way. This doesn't mean not sharing and
asking for support and guidance from others. Check in
with yourself, though; even write down what your heart
and your stomach tell you, as they often conflict. Then
see if this chimes with others. The great thing about
advice is that the right person will be suitably removed
from a situation to see the wood for the trees, so they
have more of a perspective and subjective opinion and
therefore healthy advice to give with love and compassion. This is why therapists are great.

Anger

Anger can have its roots in shame. Often from a young age we are disciplined for feeling angry, or told not to feel angry. But anger is an extremely healthy emotion to have. Anger is a motivator. Anger can enable us to mobilise. It tells us when we feel wronged.

However, there is a huge difference between anger and rage.

Many people fly into rage, which is essentially uncontrolled anger. Much like the child who throws a tantrum, adults do the same. They basically throw their toys out of the pram and, if unchecked, will do it time and time again. Rage is actually scary to behold and people can use this as a technique to get what they want.

Often it takes the greatest amount of control to stop flying into rage, or on the flip side NOT to bury one's anger. Buried anger becomes detrimental to our health. For anger doesn't just disappear – it has to be processed. If it's acted out as rage, we don't process the actual hurt, and if it's kept in, we become passive-aggressive or people-pleasers yet still have the hurt and anger bouncing around inside ourselves.

Embrace your anger. I scream into pillows, use crayons to draw it out, and exercise, especially boxing or kickboxing. Use that power. The shamans (see page 164) embrace the jaguar especially as an animal that can be unleashed to protect us.

Animals

Animals have the most wonderful sense of 'being'. Animals simply exist. They live to eat, sleep, procreate and, in some cases, receive and give affection. An animal's nervous system needs to be settled all of the time to allow it to preserve its fight-or-flight responses when needs be. Horses are a wonderful example of this. This is why horse therapy is so fantastic. Sitting among horses can give a sense of pure calm and of being at one. They are completely present animals because they have to be. The herd constantly has to be settled to maintain its reserves in case there is a true emergency. Pack animals maintain this necessary balance of 'calm yet ready'. Like a martial artist, they are grounded and present and therefore maintain a deep power to GO if needs be.

We are fight-or-flight animals and therefore need our nervous systems to be settled. Animals can often do this. They literally settle our bodies with their bodies and energy. Quite remarkable really.

I do not recommend trying this with an angry llama (true story). Most animals, however, luckily don't chase you around a field, biting your bottom.

Anxiety

Now this is a HUGE topic. We feel anxious about many things, so I am going to split this into two categories:

- Real-life present-day events
- Past triggered anxiety

When I say real-life present-day events, what I mean by this is basic tangible things. For example ... I am anxious about a job interview, I am anxious about my son starting his new school, I am anxious about my wife's behaviour when we go out for dinner, etc.

These are things that I say can be checked out. So, if I am anxious about a job interview, what's the worst-case scenario and HOW bad would this be? Is it life or death? Will my health be affected? What can I tangibly do about the worst-case scenario if I don't get the job – if I can't afford my rent and have to move out, what would I do? Once you have the answers to these questions, THEN solve the problem. Rather than create fake catastrophes, this process enables me to look at what I am actually scared of and have a plan in place to solve the potential worst-case problem. The brain likes to solve problems; it is designed to do this. So let it. What this does for me is take away the anxiety of the actual occasion or circumstances that are presenting themselves for I realise it isn't that actual thing that worries me but potential consequences. The great thing as well is that my brain can then see that these things HAVEN'T happened yet so I can then focus on what is occurring in the here and now.

Sometimes anxiety is brought on by events that happened in our past. So, if I am worrying about my boy going to school for the first time and my emotional reaction is way off the Richter scale then it is likely some of my own past stuff has been triggered. A technique that helps me assess this is to look past the actual events that are worrying me and 'float' my body back to a time when I've felt these emotions before. In fact, my rule for any inflated emotions is always that I could be triggered by some past stuff. Perhaps with my son, his first day at school is triggering my own anxiety of going to school for the first time. These emotions have come flooding back to me so I am effectively 'back in that place'. I will be experiencing exactly the same emotions I felt at five years old en route to school in my mum's Ford Escort, almost feeling like I am physically there. Once I identify this I instantly relax and can then deal with the present concerns.

Here is an example. I gave someone an option: they could choose one of two Christmas jumpers I'd bought in a second-hand clothes shop. The person loved one of them. An hour later they came back, saying they couldn't stop worrying that they hadn't given the second jumper a chance. They were overly worried about it. I kept on asking the person why they were worried and this is how the conversation went:

'Why are you worried about not giving the other jumper a chance?'

'I'm anxious I've made the wrong decision.'

'And why would this worry you?'

'Er ... because if I've made the wrong decision, I've made a mistake.'

'And why are you anxious about making a mistake?'

'Because if I make a mistake, I've let someone down.'

'And why are you anxious about letting someone down?'

'Because then I'm in trouble and a bad person.'

We very quickly got to the root of the person's anxiety, which actually had nothing to do with the jumpers whatsoever and rather was about past triggered emotions around not being good enough. This technique of digging deeper by constantly asking why is a wonderful cognitive tool that I use all the time.

So, to summarise, we can experience anxiety in all forms and for all reasons. Cognitive behavioural therapy, or CBT (see page 41), can help a lot for this. Digging deeper into past triggered emotions sitting behind the anxiety is both tough and rewarding. However, it shouldn't be entered into lightly or without additional support in place.

I recommend any ways to calm the body down, be they exercise, acupuncture, massage, cranial osteopathy, a foot rub, a hot water bottle and a blanket ... To calm the body calms the mind.

Appropriate

'Appropriate' is such a wonderful fulcrum upon which to centre so many of our thoughts, intentions, words and actions. It is a word that I think has got a lot more attention over the last few years and rightfully so. To me, judging whether something is appropriate or not requires us to take a situation – either at work or out of work – and look at it through the simple lens of 'Is this right or wrong within this context?' Knowing what we find inappropriate and appropriate allows us to bolster our self-confidence and maintain our self-esteem. It shows what we will and won't tolerate. For example, I simply will not condone shouting as appropriate. I also think an inordinate amount of swearing is not appropriate in the workplace. For me, these are two things that are not appropriate working conditions and are things I feel neither I nor the people I work with should be faced with.

Arguments

I don't have many arguments. I have discussions, but honestly I see no need for an argument. They are heated, normally meaning that both sides have lost control, and they can very quickly turn to nastiness and name calling. Never bring people's friends or families into an argument when you are a couple. It is what my brother used to call 'low blows'. If it is about one or more members of that group, own YOUR feelings in it and how you feel and don't look to throw them under the bus. We must respect the relationships that our partner has with others and the history and context of those relationships.

Never insult or put down your partner in public, for example, publicly shaming at the dinner table: 'Oh well, Jonny never cooks for me'. It is bad form and shows a lack of loyalty. It happens so often and it is always a sign to me of a partner looking to garner support for their hurt feelings. It is understandable yet disloyal, and never works out.

The key to having a discussion is to own our own feelings. Don't stray from the pronoun 'I'. Years ago, my neighbour came over in a fluster because a drain was leaking that ran under my garden into theirs. The person started the conversation with 'Well, what are WE going to do about it?' I immediately stopped her and asked for what I call a 'vulnerable request'; it is essentially a polite ask. 'Can I vulnerably request that you stick to the word "I" in this conversation, please, because I don't see a WE in this situation.'

It stopped the person in their tracks and it also immediately took the stress away from the situation in terms of the uncontained anxiety that was being thrown my way. My neighbour needed to own their own feelings and not subconsciously bring me into this grouping of stress!

Pronouns are ESSENTIAL to prevent discussions moving into argument territory.

Another example is when I was doing a theatre show called *Cabaret*. At the beginning of each performance, I would appear through a little circle cut into the scenery hanging down to cover the whole front of the stage. Essentially from the outside it looked like a camera lens opening, through which I poked my little clown-like face. The music at the beginning was very quiet and people would talk in the wings, which would make it hard for me to hear the music and therefore perform the song. I had asked a few times through the correct channels that people remain quiet and yet it persisted. I was just learning to set boundaries and so despite there being a set hierarchy in place through which people could air their grievances I decided I'd had enough! I asked the company if people could kindly be quiet and said I felt scared and disrespected when I couldn't hear the music and that what I wished for was silence because it was particularly hard to hear at that moment in the show.

Afterwards a company member came into my dressing room and said that she felt extremely disrespected and that others felt the same. She felt told off and that it had not been done in the proper way. Every time that the company member would start saying herself 'and others', I would stop her and ask if she could just speak for herself and not others because, one, they weren't present and, two, if it was a few people feeling this then I suggested a company meeting so people could voice their opinions. I had to ask a couple of times for my colleague and friend to stick to using the pronoun 'I' and eventually it transpired that she felt triggered and never reacted well to feeling told off because of past stuff, which I completely validated.

Often people will look to bring others into an argument – others who aren't even present – which leads to a huge imbalance. It is not fair or correct to, say, bring something up with a friend and say, 'Well, it isn't just me, a lot of us feel you are ...' It creates an atmosphere of being ganged up on, and people will use this method when they find it hard to validate their own responses and feelings and aren't confident in themselves. Often this will lead to conflict. Make sure that both sides of a discussion maintain the 'I' position; otherwise, it very quickly turns into an argument.

People often think that arguments in the workplace are OK, but they aren't. There is never a reason, really, to have an argument. The problem is that we so often see a modelling of certain behaviours by our bosses or other colleagues that we believe it is OK to be a certain way at work. It isn't (see more on Work on page 181).

B

Being Present

I will admit I get irritated sometimes by the phrase 'let's get into the present', and the truth is it's probably because I can find it rather difficult to do, especially if I am feeling heavily anxious. That being said, I have learnt that the simple exercise of it and the repetition is calming and actually rather wonderful. It has had knock-on effects I didn't expect.

So, what is 'being in the present' and how do we do it? Being in the present is focusing purely on the moment, not thinking of the past or the future. Being in the present is not always easy and so comes with no expectations that turn into frustration and self-shaming. There are simple tools to get into the present and these are useful because often when we get triggered or are worrying it takes us out of the current moment. The shaman Jo Bowlby talks of using the five senses. Check in with what you can hear: what sound is the furthest away and what is the nearest? What can you see? Again, what is the nearest and what is the furthest away? What can you smell? What can you taste, and finally what can you feel? It's actually quite a fun thing to do and I have found if I enter into this exercise with that sense of fun, I don't tend to look to get anything too heavy out of it. It is a clever tool because it can be used anywhere and it is a good grounding tool.

We as humans don't tend to be in the present that much. Animals live beautifully in the present. They eat, play, sleep, walk, sometimes make babies and get stroked. Getting into the present allows us to see what we can choose to hold on to and what we can let go of. Being in the present can bring up a huge amount of gratitude the more you practise it. Gratitude, I believe, can make us feel happier and at peace more deeply. Right now I am grateful for the jumper I'm wearing, my laptop, my legs and my lungs. It is another great way of getting present. The trick is don't pressure yourself. Just do little things and then notice after a while what changes might have happened. You might surprise yourself.

Biased Thinking

Biased thinking is something that is very much attached to CBT – cognitive behavioural therapy (see page 41). I must say biased thinking really has been very useful and the more I tuned into my thinking and became mindful of it, using exercises from CBT, the more it became second nature to always do what I call 'checking in' with my thought processes, which is where I ask myself 'How useful is this thought right now?'

There is a plethora of biased thinking categories and essentially it involves looking at how our thoughts can view things through a prism of negativity. By exploring and observing our thoughts, we can learn to avoid reverting to patterns of thinking that set us up for a road to nowhere.

Body Image

I've always had some sort of body image shame knocking around. Sometimes it's worse than other times. I like to talk about it because it's something that I feel has been put onto me by the modern world. I recognise it as a completely external pressure and force that has internalised within me. People can suffer greatly from body image difficulties and this can lead to body dysmorphia, which is when a person feels they are in the wrong body, almost like an alien in their own skin. It can lead to people focusing on body parts and having a completely overblown and fixated view of them.

I believe the key with body image is to first notice what messages are coming from one's external world, like advertising and social media, and limit one's exposure to them. It can be damaging, and an important thing to remember is the more miserable people feel about themselves, the more likely they are to spend money. If we all felt we looked perfect as we were, we wouldn't go out to buy that new jumper to look like David Beckham, for example … It's a clever advertising tactic to shame or cajole: companies put out aspirational, unrealistic images that are never attainable. Cut it out of your life. Check who you follow on social media and check in with how you actually feel after you've seen a post of theirs; if you don't feel great, don't follow them. Every few weeks I check who I'm following and why and then do a cull. Not as a personal vendetta to the person or brand I'm following but as a way of keeping myself on track. This includes following very good-looking men with six-packs and porcelain skin. It's not their fault they look like that or choose to make money out of it; it's my reaction to them that is mostly damaging for me. I follow puppies, flowers, gardens, designers and try to cut out people who seem to portray these perfect lifestyles. They just make me feel shit and I own that.

Body Work

There is a wonderful book called *The Body Keeps the Score* by Bessel van der Kolk. The title encapsulates a lot in a few words. Unfortunately, body treatment and the way of allowing the body to show us what is going on is very much dismissed by the majority as a hippie-like approach. The reality is that body treatment is very much rooted in science.

Often our nervous systems can get activated and they can drive our minds. We think of this being the other way round and it is true: thoughts can drive emotions. It is also true, however, that the basic primal reactions of fight, flight or freeze within the body can and will drive the mind to search for a solution, and unfortunately this can create problems. For example, if I am trying to go to sleep but my body is in a state of heightened anxiety, my mind might decide that I must completely repaint my bedroom. If I were to follow through on this, I would be allowing my mind to run the show and not be listening to my body. The key here is to listen to the body and act accordingly. Instead of painting, I would lie on the floor, allowing my back to feel the support beneath it. I'm therefore showing my body that it is safe. My body calms down and I save a lot in paint. In fact, for any moment, if we have a calm body and our nervous system is working peacefully, then anything can be dealt with in a composed, more relaxed way.

Here are my recommendations for calming the body:

- Acupuncture is a practice used in traditional Chinese medicine. Acupuncturists insert thin needles into the skin at specific points around the body to balance your energy and help target specific areas that need healing. It's very good for releasing tension. I think it's a wonderful experience; it's just the fear of needles that is the tough bit for some of us!
- Cranial osteopathy is a type of osteopathic treatment where the practitioner applies gentle pressure to the head and spine to encourage the release of stresses throughout the body. It can be used to treat a range of health issues and is also extremely relaxing and amazing for enabling good sleep.
- Going to see an osteopath or physiotherapist or having a massage are all good ways of relaxing the body, but baths, showers, gentle stretching and even dancing are other simple things you can do at home. Tai chi and yoga are other gentle ways.

Try any of these things and see how you feel before and then afterwards. When our body is settled and relaxed, our mind is also likely to be more settled and we are able to see things more clearly. How do we know when our body is settled? We move from a state of doing to a state of being and feel very little is troubling us.

Bosses

How do we deal with challenging bosses? It's a hard one. Often we can work under people who are difficult. They enjoy their power and enjoy shaming people in front of others. Bosses often withhold praise, which is another way of maintaining what they perceive as power. How do we handle an unpleasant boss, perhaps one that is passive-aggressive and actually acts as a defunct adult child? It's so difficult because we need to earn money; we have the pressures of ensuring our own financial safety and that for our families if we have children.

An abusive boss can tap into and trigger our very core feelings of safety because we need to earn to look after our basic needs of shelter and food and water.

There are several routes we can take in dealing with a difficult boss. We can go to HR if things seem really bad and of course if there is an HR department available. If the boss is completely inappropriate and abusive, we can go to tribunals. We can try feeding back to a boss; however, I would suggest if one's boss is too far gone in terms of an inability to have any emotional awareness, you might not feel safe doing this. We can start to look for other jobs while remaining in our present one.

Write up your various areas of your life on a piece of paper and then make sure to ring-fence each one. It shows that we are more than just our work. Make sure you get resourced and enriched from the other areas of your life. Make sure you remain boundaried. If I am in a toxic work environment, I imagine a jaguar standing in front of the people I find intolerable. In meetings, I often place the jaguar on the table right in front of me! Practise staying rooted and, when interacting with your boss, remain grounded: focus on your breathing and remind yourself you are incredible.

Ultimately, though, if it is too intolerable and you are able to … get the hell out of there.

Boundaries

I mean, this really is one of the BIG topics in wellbeing. It is the equivalent of the Big Five African wildlife (lion, leopard, elephant, rhino and buffalo).

So, animals aside, here we go. I split boundaries into three categories: the physical boundary, the imagined/ emotionally protective boundary and the spoken boundary.

1 The physical boundary is literally how close you would want someone to you. So many times, people violate our physical boundaries. This can be by standing too close, coming in for a hug when you haven't actually asked for one, or touching you, which then stretches to overtly sexual behaviour when this is not actually what is wanted. The key here is to recognise how important our body and our physical space is to us. For example, a few years ago, I was waiting for a drink at the bar in my local pub. I noticed another customer come in and even though it was just me standing at the bar, they decided to plonk themselves about fifteen centimetres away from my left arm. To me, this felt uncomfortable and not the appropriate amount of distance I wanted between myself and a stranger. I decided to gently move myself about half a metre to my right for my own sense of personal space. What was fascinating was that the person quite subconsciously moved the same distance closer to me.

I realised that this person clearly had some issues with physical boundaries, so I asked the barman to hold my drink behind the bar while I went to use the restroom, hence alleviating the problem of the clingy customer and lack of physical boundary.

2 The imagined boundary I call the suit of armour. Every day I imagine my suit of armour (mine is a Batman suit ... I love it) about fifty times a day. It enables me to not take on other people's stuff and also protect myself when people are giving their opinions on my work, my clothes, the fact I'm wearing a hat, and, weirdly, the fact that I am wearing glasses to 'disguise' myself. (For the record, if I don't wear glasses I can't see.) Around this suit I then have a wider, extended imagined boundary. Sometimes I cannot cope with people's energies. This is normally when a person is emotionally uncontained (see page 68) and it just seeps out of their pores. With some people I actually imagine they are a football pitch away from me and, if I really am getting a vibe that I don't like them, I physically remove myself.

3 The spoken boundary is just that – it states your needs. I actually used it yesterday. Someone said something I felt was inappropriate and I said so, said what I felt and what I would prefer. It allows us to own our feelings, discover what our true needs and wants are and gain confidence and have more self-esteem.

Breathing

It's something we all do … well, until we don't and it's time for us to depart this world. Often when we get stressed, upset, angry or experience any heightened emotion, we can forget to breathe properly. We begin to take more shallow breaths. There is an anatomical reason for this – as animals, the taking of more shallow breaths gets cortisol and adrenaline rushing round our bodies. This prepares us for a basic instinct of fight, flight or freeze. This was fine when we were cavemen, yet not so useful when we are having a disagreement with our partner! Hopefully, stone hammers aren't to hand.

By concentrating on our breathing, slowing it down and thinking about receiving the breath in our lungs, we can in turn calm our body. This allows us to approach what is going on in a calmer and more measured manner.

Breathing is a huge topic and there is lots of fascinating research into how breathing correctly affects our physical and mental wellbeing. I highly recommend a fantastic book about breathing by James Nestor called *Breath*. He has gone back through centuries of ancient wisdom to look at how the way we breathe has changed and how breathing the right way can help our health, our mind and our nervous system and even help cure conditions such as asthma.

But

Years ago I went on a week-long course to do with love avoidance and addiction. I wasn't really in the space to properly take on board what was being said, and to be honest I didn't gel with the guy who ran it, but the best thing I learnt was the use of the word 'BUT' and replacing it with 'AND'. It seems such a tiny thing and it is actually massive.

Let's dissect this sentence: 'I feel really sad today and extremely anxious, BUT it's OK, I am getting by.'

The first half of the sentence is an open exclamation of my feelings and the second half is saying I am getting by with my day. Placing 'BUT' in the middle presents a fulcrum upon which the context of the sentence hinges. It discredits my feelings as a negative thing: 'I'm feeling this, BUT ...'

Let's look at the sentence with the use of the word 'AND': 'I feel really sad today and extremely anxious, AND it's OK, I am getting by.'

Do you notice how using 'AND' instead of 'BUT' as the hinging point sets no negative connotation onto my feelings? My feelings are my feelings. We use 'BUT' so many times. Even when writing my sentence above earlier, I was going to say, 'It seems a tiny thing but it is actually massive.'

What 'AND' does is allow a neutral flow. We so often, by using the word 'BUT', discredit our own words. I urge you to recognise when you use the word and replace it with 'AND' and see how you feel. It can feel uncomfortable at first because we aren't used to fully claiming and owning our words, thoughts and feelings *and* it really, really works!

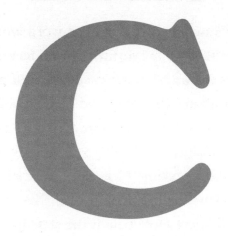

Catastrophising

This is when we think in an extreme manner and predict the very worst. For example, I heard a friend say, after they broke up with their partner, 'Well, I will NEVER find a boyfriend now, I will NEVER have a child now, the WHOLE thing was a complete waste of time.'

It is important to state here that sometimes I think therapists or certain books can move to invalidate these feelings. For me, it is essential we still validate these thoughts and feelings. We should never shame ourselves for our thoughts; we can, however, observe, be curious and explore a new way of thinking.

'Should be' statements

We can berate ourselves by using the word 'should'. As soon as I notice I have 'should' in my mind or vocabulary,

I stop myself and check it out, asking, 'How useful is this to me? Why SHOULD I do anything?' The word imposes expectations and usually leads me down a self-blaming and self-shaming dead end.

A very good little technique I like to use with my thoughts and which can apply to all these types of biased thinking is fact-checking. How true is the statement that I SHOULD be far more successful, that I SHOULD have more money? How true is the statement that I will NEVER meet a partner and NEVER find happiness? That EVERYONE hates me and I have NO friends at all? It's a really useful way of taking the heat out of one's thoughts and keeping them from spiralling.

CBT

CBT stands for cognitive behavioural therapy. It is a therapy that looks at what we are doing and produces exercises for us to work at and aids in improving our lifestyle. It is an analysis, but also looks at how we can let our brain work for us. Currently, the NHS tends to offer up to twenty sessions, and further support is available if needed. If you refer yourself via IAPT (Improving Access to Psychological Therapies), you are often offered six sessions, then a further referral if necessary. Still, this is something we can do on our own. It takes time and it takes persistence and it does work, believe me. I worked with a CBT-based therapist for a while and it helped a lot with my social anxiety, nerves around speaking in public, etc. What you put in is what you get out of it. It is the gym for our minds and can really help us get through life and navigate the way our minds can work.

There are many 'traps' that CBT shows our brains can fall into, and by highlighting these it allows us to take a breath and aim to slowly be able to make better choices in our thinking. For example, black-and-white thinking – or all-or-nothing thinking, as it is also known – is one area where our mind can go to a place of believing complete totalitarianism when we look at our lives:

'I will NEVER work again.'

'I will NEVER meet a partner.'

'I NEVER have any fun.'

'ALL my friends hate me.'

These are self-beliefs that we can look at, notice we are exaggerating and then look to unpick.

Catastrophising is another unuseful thinking trap where we will take something to the extreme. For example, I'm running late, and I think that I won't get my child to school and then I'll be late for work as well, then I think that my child will be expelled and that I will lose my job … It is going to the absolute worst-case scenario when there isn't any evidence that this is going to happen.

We can also fall into the traps of comparing ourselves to others, or trying to be the perfectionist. Highlighting these types of thought patterns with CBT allows us to take a step back and ask ourselves, 'How useful is this thinking and is there a better way to approach life in my mind?'

Children

You have to know yourself to have kids, is my thought process. If we don't know ourselves, how will we know what we are being like around our kids? To parent is an amazing thing because it gets our adult on board. I'm not saying have kids to ensure you are constantly in your adult; however, remember to ask yourself in the moment, 'Am I being the adult or the child?'

So often we engage with our children in conflict on the same wavelength as them. What I mean by this is you might as well put two thirteen-year-olds in a ring and let them slug it out. It's a lose-lose battle. Remember YOU ARE THE PARENT and even during times when you react – because you are not impervious to stress, hurt, annoyances, etc. – remember you cannot stoop to the level of your child. You must maintain the appropriate boundaries, appropriate communication and appropriate actions that are required of a parent.

If your child talks back and suddenly you talk back to them, what good does this do? If your child insults you and you insult them back, what is this showing them? Always ask yourself, 'What am I showing my kids in this moment?' It's not easy and it shouldn't be about shaming yourself. Also, if you have not had the best modelling from your parents on how to bring up a child, it's going to be tough. It is, however, essential. Work on your communication, work on your ability to express your feelings and love to your children. Create a unit; become a family unit where everyone works for each other.

Manners ... they are essential. Remember to ask yourself, 'Am I asking stuff from my children that I don't do myself? If I'm expecting good manners, am I modelling good manners to them?'

It's bloody hard and I know only what I observe and have learnt. I don't judge at all because when you are handling washing, cooking and cleaning as well as disciplining and ferrying kids around, it's not easy. Don't be afraid to ask for help. No parent is perfect and we all need help.

Christmas

So, Christmas. I am going out on a limb and saying it is the most REACTIVE of times. Any old family systems (see page 90) in place will rear up like an old shadow. Aged forty-three, I still occasionally go back to being the people-pleaser, isolating in my bedroom and watching the *EastEnders* omnibus. I'm using Christmas as an example here as it relates to my own experience but the same thoughts can be applied to any family gatherings or holidays in general.

I was wondering why Christmas is often such a fraught time for families, and I think it's because it's become a sort of focal point of how 'together' a family should be and how dysfunctional it actually is. The pressure of forced fun, beautiful family engagement and perfect scenes of laughter and love that is reinforced through advertising creates an expectation that is totally unrealistic for most families. The interesting thing to me is that Christmas has been completely hijacked from being a religious festival to something that serves capitalism perfectly. Even Father Christmas has been co-opted by mass marketing; he was green until Coca-Cola changed him to red for their own ad campaigns! It sort of sums up Christmastime, doesn't it? Anyway, the problem is that this sense of expectation puts into glaring focus the dysfunctions of any given family. If it were any other day, there would be more acceptance –

or at the least, less of a juxtaposition between the feigned notion of what Christmas *should* be and the realistic complication of getting a family together at any time of year. So, remember: Christmas is actually just another day. When you can see it as that, it makes it far less heightened.

Here are a few more tips to get through it:

1 My old therapist told me a quick Christmas is the best Christmas. In other words, get in and get OUT. By giving yourself a time frame it can settle the younger parts of you that will get activated by allowing them to see that they are not going back to that way of living and they have a choice whether to go or stay.

2 Once you have in place the allotted time you will spend with your family at Christmas it is time to practise empathy. Think of what your parents and siblings had to grow up with. After all, family systems and dynamics are often down to learnt behaviour they observed in their own parents. Practising empathy and understanding allows you to let go of the behaviours that might unfold around you, perhaps forgiving some of the barbed comments that could usually trigger old feelings.

3 Keep in touch with people in your life who represent a new family, like friends or partners who validate you and accept you for who you are. They will keep you grounded in the here and now.

4 Try not to drink too much. Alcohol can be a good settler, but it can also make you let go of your defences. I'm not saying don't enjoy yourself, but better to enjoy yourself when you feel completely safe and in a nurturing environment.

5 Practise goodwill and giving by helping others. Visit sick people in hospital, bring meals to people who don't have company or are unable to cook for themselves, or help homeless charities. Often people will criticise these things as being disingenuous. No. Helping people while also helping yourself is completely natural and is, after all, why people help people. It is about true connection and practising love. By being kind to others, of course you are bound to feel kinder towards yourself. This isn't some sort of Darwinian hooded cloak of selfishness; it is actually tapping into true love and understanding and compassion – themes that are central to Christmas. The creation of a day that should seemingly be the 'happiest day ever' creates a whole vacuum of sadness and loneliness, and to aid in filling that is a wonderful and fulfilling thing. Embrace it.

Cleaning

I absolutely love cleaning! I don't have OCD (a compulsion to clean is a common symptom of clinical OCD) and I don't obsessively clean and yet I do notice that a tidy home leads to a tidy mind. There is a famous speech from Navy SEAL Admiral William H. McRaven that was doing the rounds a few years ago. The speech rallied on the importance of making one's bed first thing in the morning. Such a small thing and it does really make a difference. It shows discipline and preparedness for the day and I have found it shifts something in me, however small. I widen this out to one's whole house. To love and nurture one's home is to show pride and respect and – again, that word – gratitude. To look after your house and keep it clean shows an outward sense of pride and care and I have really enjoyed nurturing my house over the last few years. It is always a sign for me that I am off-track when my home becomes messy and dishevelled.

Clothes

I actually think clothes are so fundamental in many ways. Use clothes in the right way and they become the most useful tool. Clothes are not about what is in fashion, or what others think, or fitting in, or using them to shame yourself for your size. Clothes are about celebrating, literally dressing up, creating, enjoying, playing and role-playing! People have so many different approaches to clothes. What is key, though, is that if you don't feel comfortable in a piece of clothing, don't wear it: simple. If you don't feel comfortable, the clothes will wear you.

This being said, try pushing yourself out of your comfort zone just to see what happens. A certain skirt might feel a bit racy to begin with, but that may be because you aren't used to feeling sexy, so check it out. Wear it to the shops and see how you feel. It is a balance and you never want to be someone you aren't. People don't marry your clothes, fall in love with your clothes, ask your clothes out for coffee. Clothes are there to be enjoyed and act as supports for you. Don't take them too seriously. Mix and match from charity shops to designers. Shop in only the sales for designer stuff is my tip, especially online. Get one good coat, one good suit, one good pair of shoes and several good T-shirts! Always play around. See how much you don't need them, see how much you can use them.

I went away once for two months with only a back-pack and I didn't find myself thinking, *God, I miss my clothes.* In fact, the stress of not having to look at what I wore that day was wonderful. I have a friend who only wears white T-shirts, black trousers, a dark grey hoodie, one black jacket and one black jumper and always the same shoes. He does it as he says it takes a lot of stress out of his life. I love it.

Play around. Never feel trapped by your clothes. Throw away the ones you don't fit into anymore rather than constantly staring at them, thinking, *God, I wish I was thinner.* Let others use them.

Co-Dependency

Co-dependency is quite a difficult topic to define, so let me start by recommending a book by Pia Mellody called *Facing Codependence*. Pia writes and talks very succinctly about co-dependency and outlines a framework for identifying co-dependent thinking, behaviour and emotions.

Essentially, co-dependency occurs where we have an imbalanced relationship in which one person has an unhealthy reliance on someone else. My wellbeing and peace rely on, or are sacrificed for, someone else, be that a boss, sibling, parent, friend or partner.

This sense of reliance can come out in a number of behaviours. It can make us people-pleasers, fixers, enablers; ensuring that as long as someone else's needs are looked after, our own needs don't matter. It can also make us manipulators. I was always desperate to be 'nice Will Young' so would modify my true self and feelings and behaviour to make someone like me. It is a form of manipulation and can make me conceal my true thoughts and feelings.

For example, if a friend upset me at a dinner by insulting the food I cooked (this would rarely happen as I don't really like cooking and rarely have people round to my house!) and I simply let this insult and my hurt feelings go because I didn't want to seem nasty and lose that friendship, I would essentially be presenting a false representation of myself simply to maintain my image of being jovial and nice. Or let's say I am let down by a friend at the last minute when they, for the third time, don't turn up to my birthday, and I say, 'Oh, don't worry, it is absolutely fine', while actually holding on to huge amounts of anger and upset underneath. I am again being dishonest and ultimately not experiencing an honest friendship. In both of these examples, my fear of rejection is so innate and I am so co-dependent that I let people walk all over me and in turn build up mounds of residual anger inside that can make me ill.

We are all born co-dependent. When we are babies, toddlers, children and even progressing young adults, we are dependent on a parental figure – the other – to ensure that our basic needs and wants are met. If there is any risk to our needs being met and our safety assured, we as humans, children and even babies are extremely resourceful and will adapt our behaviour to ensure we get noticed, we get fed, we get the attention and love we need. Over time these behaviours can turn maladaptive and lead to a type of co-dependence in later life that is not healthy. We remain stuck in this maladaptive cycle of behaviour and role-playing and may become a perfectionist, trying to be the perfect person who is nice to everyone.

At its genesis, co-dependence is nothing other than an essential and obvious situation where to get our needs met we HAD to rely on another human being. When we deal with the base of our adult co-dependency

– interrogating how our needs in earlier years weren't met and what we are still pining for and trying to set right – we gain an understanding and compassion for our own co-dependent tendencies.

Mine, for example, is still to please my mother even if it is to my detriment. I have to watch myself like a hawk to ensure I practise self-care. Sometimes I trip up and that's OK because I have overall self-love and under-standing for the genesis of my co-dependent behaviours around my mother. The best thing is that, now that I keep an eye on myself, my relationship with my mother is so much better!

I can also feel it generally with friends and even work colleagues. If my brother isn't settled then I can't be settled. I understand this and also try my hardest to own and understand my own emotions so I can be truly pres-ent for others. There is even a twelve-step program called 'CoDA' (Co-Dependents Anonymous), which helps people to process and express their emotional states.

I worry sometimes that co-dependency can become an extremely shaming thing when we are pushed the whole time to be an island, to just love ourselves from within and rely on no one else, maintaining boundaries. Of course we need this; however, I also believe we need a level of co-dependency in the healthiest of relationships. It is about striking a balance, so a level of neediness is not a bad thing; it just allows us to rely on our partner, the key being the choosing of said partner and existing within the realms of a healthy, non-toxic relationship. We are allowed to have needs and look to get those met from a partner, as long as our happiness doesn't solely depend on someone else, and I think sometimes the expectation to completely avoid co-dependency within a certain therapeutic community can be damaging and unrealistic.

Coming Out

It is often said that LGBTQIA+ people have to constantly come out for the rest of their lives. Heterosexual people don't need to constantly declare who they are sexually attracted to, and cisgender people don't need to tell everybody about their gender identity. For this section I've chosen to speak about coming out as a gay man but I am aware it can be very different for other members of the LGBTQIA+ community.

Coming out is really a bit unfair. I mean, I think declaring at the kitchen table that you just don't like liver and will never eat it again is fine and, gosh, who knows, could create a bit of a conflict within the family. Telling my grandfather that I just do not and will not ever like lawn bowls, as painful as it was for him to hear from his grandson, he got over it. If being gay could be in that category of everyday acknowledgements of likes and dislikes, then hoorah, wouldn't the world be great? But even though things are so much better today and it is far more of a non-event for many societies, 'coming out' is still a big deal. This is largely because of the history of shame associated with being gay that a young person will have absorbed throughout their life, so when they discover they are themselves gay, they are made to feel defunct and different and freakish. Coming out isn't an empowering declaration of one's desires in all cases; rather it can feel like an admission of a crime of thought and lust. In certain papers it will still be written, 'So-and-so ADMITS to being gay', as if it is some sort of seedy wrong secret.

Because of all the shame heaped on homosexuality through all sorts of mediums, we are terrified of what the repercussions will be of coming out. These can be reinforced by families' reactions. When I came out, my mother said she was worried I would be beaten up and taken advantage of and go on gay marches. My friend was told he was going to grow old and die alone, while a former boyfriend's mum said, 'What will we tell the neighbours?' Sometimes, when the parent loves their child deeply, they are driven by that love to say the most inappropriate and unhelpful things. I remember saying to my mother that being told I was going to be beaten up wasn't the most heart-warming notion after years of feeling muted and unable to express I was gay. Worse than these reactions, though, is when a parent is worried about themselves and not their child. To come out is to leave yourself open to anything negative, ranging from ridicule to the risk of death. The spectrum unfortunately is that wide.

Coming out doesn't stop with parents and families; it also involves friends and then people in the workplace. At every level, the implications of risk and unwanted attention have to be considered. I know people that are out to friends, yet not out at work or to their parents:

damage limitation. I don't judge this. However, what I have observed in myself is that the more open I am about myself (though not necessarily shouting it from the rooftops), the more pride I have in myself. Perhaps coming out twenty times a day, every single day, has helped me to come out with my simpler needs and my wants:

'No, thanks, I don't want mayonnaise with my fries.'

'No, I don't have a wife; I have a husband.'

'I like that jumper, but if you don't have any more orange ones I am not interested, thank you.'

The declarations we can make to the world about ourselves are endless, and so I like to see coming out as part of that and look at it as reminding me to celebrate myself every minute of every day.

Commitment

Firstly, I would like to mention The Commitments, a fictional nineties band who aren't necessarily anything to do with wellbeing but are a very good group to listen to.

COMMITMENT ... now this can feel like a big word, and I guess it is. What does the idea of commitment bring up for the individual? For me, it brings up a sense of purpose, being committed to a cause, as well as committed to my core values. It is a pact and a sign of trust and protectiveness and self-belief – for me to be committed to myself and who I believe I am and what my needs and wants are, and how I expect to treat others and be treated. Commitment in a relationship can bring up a sense of feeling trapped, unable to escape, claustrophobic and scared, worried about the other person: 'What if I hurt them? What if I can't deliver?' Alternatively, it can bring up our fears of abandonment: 'What if they leave me? How will I cope?'

As well as relationships, I extend this to being socially committed to friends and occasions. I often don't like saying I will do something. I don't like fully committing to a dinner or a party or even a wedding. I feel trapped again and like I can't get out of it, and what happens if I really don't want to see people that day and I'm feeling anxious? I don't want to commit to things as I feel unsafe and ungrounded and like I have lost my base. I cannot find my safety in social situations. In this way I find committing to actually turning up to things difficult. (For tips on what to do in this situation and how to handle it, see Party Nerves on page 150.)

Commitment can also be a positive thing – for example, I think of commitment to my family and my nieces and nephews; I am committed to ensuring they are heard and listened to by me and all their needs from emotional to physical to spiritual wellbeing are observed by me and aided and nurtured to the best of my ability. I am fully committed to this.

I have been fully committed to my mental and physical health, and commitment was one of the things that got me through being so unwell and pushed me through my treatment when so often I wanted to give up.

Commitment is very underestimated in its meaning and its effect. It shows loyalty, trust, determination, doggedness, stubbornness and protectiveness and allows for connectivity. It is something that is ever moving forward and forever needing to be reinforced, and it will be forever tested and challenged, both externally and internally.

Communication

Communication is key. It sounds so obvious, but it is of course true, and we so often forget to communicate. By definition, communication is the imparting or exchanging of information through speaking, writing or some other medium. It allows a person to seek or provide information and to share their emotions or feelings. I believe the best type of communication is clear, concise and consistent.

In relationships, so often a breakdown of communication is at the root of conflict and angst. If I think about it in basic terms, if I forget to tell my partner that I am getting milk and he gets milk as well then we have two lots of fresh milk, meaning one might end up going off. We tend to not forget these things, yet we can forget to communicate our feelings to each other. This spreads across all relationships, friendships, families and business environments.

One time I had a set-to with a friend. I was feeling that they weren't making an effort to come and see me or check in on me while I was in treatment for anxiety. It was a huge projection on my behalf and my reaction was overinflated; however, there was a good moment between myself and the friend. She said that she had actually had a health scare recently so there was stuff going on in HER life that I didn't realise. What I said was how was I to know if she, as one of my best friends, wasn't actually telling me of these things?

What are blocks to communication? Lack of consistency might be one. It is not a one-time thing; it has to be continuous. Think of a business; communication must be continual so things run like a well-oiled machine.

A block might be a lack of the necessary environment where communication is encouraged and nurtured. There is no point in attempting to have a continual dialogue if one side isn't at all interested in listening or the atmosphere is not one of respect and support.

It is also important to communicate in a respectful and calm manner. Often I write things down to help with this.

A final thing to ask oneself is, 'Am I getting frustrated about things that perhaps I haven't even openly disclosed to the other party?' Is it reasonable to get continually annoyed at my neighbours' 'lack of respect' when they allow their children to scream all day and night if I don't actually communicate that I am finding it troublesome? How can I continue to take umbrage that my friend doesn't lift a finger when they come and stay if I remain silent on the matter? People are not mind-readers; WE are not mind-readers. Think – would you like to find things out about your behaviour that perhaps you are unaware of if it was upsetting a friend?

Community

I LONG for community. It has taken me a long time to allow myself to feel part of a community. Often, I felt I couldn't belong: I wasn't a good enough gay to belong to the gay community, I wasn't a good enough musician to belong to the musical community and so on and so on. I wouldn't allow myself to feel part of a community even in my local area.

To be part of a community is to feel a sense of belonging. In the West, we are now a secular society, so ties such as religion really seem to have evaporated. What I have noticed is I have a need to feel part of something. I like feeling part of my road. I like feeling part of my industry. I also like to feel part of a therapeutic community. A group that concentrates on acceptance and a place where I can be open about whatever I am feeling in that precise moment.

I have noticed how I have branched out when talking about the different types of groupings I consider to be community. It isn't just about locality or what kind of financial class we belong to or what car we drive, it is about finding our 'tribe'. It is still an ongoing thing for me and it doesn't always come easy, and I know that to feel connected and supported is an essential part of being human. Many people find a sense of community by joining an exercise group or a local organisation with shared interests, e.g. theatre, art, book clubs, etc. Taking up new hobbies is a way of finding out what you like doing and meeting like-minded people.

Conflict Resolution

I don't like the word 'conflict' in this context. It's not that I am afraid of conflict, I just don't think it is the right word to describe two people coming to a place where they can share what they are thinking and feeling and then find some resolution simply from having shared that.

To me, 'conflict resolution' immediately puts the genesis of this occurrence in a state of aggression. Perhaps my mind would be eased by thinking of conflict resolution as the decompression of a potentially highly energised interaction between two people, where no peaceful conclusion is occurring.

So ... deep breath ... conflict resolution – how can it be done? I am going to give a really obvious example of a situation where it is needed and how to get there.

I have been out to dinner and my partner felt that when I laughed as he was asking for more potatoes, I was laughing at him ordering them and shaming his appetite. When we got home my partner asked if we could speak. He deliberately did not bring it up at the dinner table or in the car but waited until we were inside the house. He owned his feelings about what I had done and it gave me the opportunity to say I hadn't heard him ordering more potatoes and I was laughing at something the person next door to me had said.

When I think of conflict resolution I like to think of laser surgery. Conflict resolution for me needs to be clean, concise and precise. We don't want a laser surgeon with a wobbly hand just as much as we don't want to let our emotions become uncontained and attacking. Keep it to YOUR stuff and YOUR experience.

Always talk from the 'I' position.

Never use the phrase 'You make me feel': no one can MAKE you feel anything. It is so crucial to own one's feelings. My god, it took me ages to realise that no one could make me feel something; it is my reaction to something that brings about the feelings. This is, of course, different to physical force and it is also not meant to undermine how cruel people can be. There might be a day, for example, when I am feeling especially grounded and strong and someone might shout an insult at me; my reaction emotionally on that day is to let it slip past me and not affect me in the slightest. In fact, sometimes I actually am just curious about why a person would be wanting to shout such things. On another day, I might be feeling particularly vulnerable and the insult will trigger crushing despair and depression. I own my emotional reaction and I work hard to not invalidate myself for whatever that is. What I will say is this is far more complex if someone is in an atmosphere of constant verbal abuse.

So, here is the format for a conversation to resolve conflict:

1. When I heard you say 'blah blah blah'
   or
   When I saw you do 'blah blah blah'
2. What came up for me was 'blah blah blah'
3. What I feel about that is [say your feeling state]
4. What I would prefer for the future is ...

This is a basic format to maintain one's sense of owner-ship and never a sense of blame or attack. I call it the Switzerland approach. The ability to take responsibil-ity for one's feelings and crucially state them in front of someone is extremely empowering. What is crucial with conflict resolution is to state what you would prefer from the future and even make a 'vulnerable request'.

I honestly use it every day and it gets easier and easier. It is crucial for me to maintain a lighter way of living where I am not carrying baggage of anger and bitterness or hurt because I get it out. There is enough of that from my past, which I find hard to own, so I might as well own the stuff in the present.

So often we do not express our anger to each other and it eats us up inside and yet we think and talk about it so much to other people that in the end we expect by osmosis that the person who has angered us SHOULD know. We forget that the crucial act of TELLING the person hasn't actually happened!

Connection

I've decided that connection is everything. We all want to feel connected and what comes with connection is a sense of feeling accepted in a group. This could be an exercise group, a Bible study group; there is also a plethora of ways to find connection through online communities. We all connect through something: a shared experience, a shared passion or a shared vulnerability. Without connection we can become islands, and the problem is that, often, if we have had problems in being let down by our caregivers in childhood, we resist connection, yet underneath we crave it.

Connection is a sense of belonging; it is a sense of safety and a sense of being needed. I have worked hard on opening my resistance to connection and honouring the felt muscle memory of not wanting to fully relax and trust connections. It has taken me a long time to see that I am OK now and connecting is a good, life-affirming thing. There are still times when I tend to isolate and can get very socially scared. A good exercise that I do is to use a CBT technique and see how I was feeling before an event and then how I felt after. I will mark my level of anxiety out of ten, with ten being the most anxious, and invariably find that I tend to feel better after the event.

Containment

This is one of my favourite words! It's not used that much and to be honest, I can't really remember when I first came across it in a wellbeing sense, but, to me, being contained is having a handle on my emotional reality at any stage of the day. If I have a handle on this it means that I can walk into a room when I might be feeling all sorts of emotions but I am validating them and recognising that I need to act appropriately, given the atmosphere I am in.

For example, as a pop star it is actually quite easy to do what I want. I hold a lot of ace cards; if I don't perform then the show doesn't happen. I'm the boss, I'm the artist, so all the stress is on me for ultimately a three-minute performance or an hour-and-a-half performance. I could think, I'm famous therefore I'm allowed to act like a complete brat and not have any containment whatsoever or emotional awareness!

By the way, I was actually like this for a bit, but was very unhappy and not very nice to be around. Lots of people are like this their whole lives and it isn't just pop stars! Anyone who is holding a position of power often doesn't bother to be contained: bosses, parents, teachers, police, etc. How often have we seen a boss explode and thought, *What the fuck are they doing*?

It is also important to think about containment at an energetic level. Some people are spilling over with uncontained anger or fear. One of my specialities is anger because I can pick it up from twenty paces due to my childhood experiences. If someone is presenting one thing but I am getting a sense of waves of uncontained anger, it freaks me out! My rule is to remove myself from a situation when I feel uncontained anger so I can feel safe.

The way we can contain our own energy is to parent ourselves and literally imagine a good boundary around our bodies, making sure that stuff is being heard and noticed but not spilling out all over the place. Never underestimate how much we as humans pick up on energy-wise; it's basic science.

Crafts

This is a great practice in mindfulness. Knitting, needle-point, colouring in, drawing, quilt making (bunting is my favourite) – all these things allow the mind to relax and focus on a very simple task at hand. Not only does it allow the body and the mind to settle, but you also end up with something at the end of it.

(For your information, my bunting sells at numerous newsagents across the south-west of the UK.)

Curiosity

One of my old therapists used to say to me when I was very ill, 'Be curious about that.' I had awful dissociation and was not functioning well at all and when she would say, 'Mm ... how curious, be curious about that.' I would reply, 'I'm finding it difficult to be constantly curious about the fact I can't see any face in the mirror!'

I actually like the phrase, though, which is why I've included something seemingly innocent. Curiosity is basically mindfulness but, in my opinion, a more empathic and interested approach. To be curious is to be engaged and to essentially care. To be curious about anything is to be open and willing to listen and be educated and learn. It's actually a wonderful approach to life to bring curiosity to everything one does. I try to be curious about people's views that I don't share or understand. Curiosity brings about love and avoids conflict and we can all get into such conflict with ourselves over how we are feeling or how we act. We can attack ourselves far worse than we would anyone else. To hang on to curiosity is to enter even just a little bit into a space of love, and so, even as I write this, it has been a welcome reminder to maintain curiosity, for others and for myself.

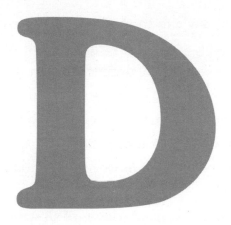

Dancing

Dancing is one of the most liberating and energy-dispersing activities. When I was younger, I was terrified about the idea of going on the dance floor. Weddings, parties or nights out, I would will myself to do it, but I felt stuck and rooted to the ground by utter self-consciousness. When I was a teenager, I would practise dancing in front of the mirror and even asked my friend who was a natural dancer to teach me. One of the main concerns was that I would look stupid. I wanted to look like a good dancer. The thing is, when kids dance, they don't give a shit! If you watch them, there is something so beautiful and authentic and joyous. As adults we lose this and get hung up on 'looking good'.

It became my aim to shake off this pre-occupation with not making a fool of myself. I started ballet lessons and my teacher spent a lot of time just getting me to walk from one corner of the dance studio to the other. I was so self-conscious even when walking. I didn't know what to do with my hands so always carried a bag or rucksack. Over time, though, I got more into my body and now I dance for joy!

Many people join dance classes of all standards, either to learn a style like salsa or hip-hop or simply to do a Zumba class! It is so good for you to learn to shake off any stress. It is natural to want to move freely; it's just our inner world that looks to restrict us. Challenge your-self and take five dance classes. Dance around your room. Dance in the dark. Depending on what your body can do, dancing will look different from one person to the next, and it is always worth exploring this form of movement as an outlet of self-expression. It's really fun and it can work to get you back into your body and change your energy state – especially if you are feeling low and shut down.

Death

It was a shaman that cured my fear of death. I say cured …
I didn't actually go looking to get over my deep fear of
death, it was for something else.

I used to have moments where, if I actually stopped
and thought about death, I began to get this paralyzing
fear. I would begin to slowly sink away, down and down,
and my mind and then body just couldn't comprehend
what death was or where I would go. I mean, how is that
possible that I could just disappear?

I am not religious, so I don't believe in heaven or
hell. The idea of eternal nothing, however, made me feel
sick. What I imagined was me in the dark, in space in
complete darkness with no one around, and with only
my consciousness, for eternity.

After visiting the shaman, what came to my mind
was that I just wouldn't be around, and, because I wasn't
around, I wouldn't know about it. There was nothing TO
experience because I wouldn't be there! Twinned with
this was an incredible sense of connection to the world
– how I would live on through life that was occurring.

People live on for me in my memory and sense of
them. The other day I finally got round to watching a
DVD my friend Jo had made for me with a BBC docu-
mentary on the ballet dancer Rudolf Nureyev. She made
it at least two years before she died. Four years later,

I finally got round to watching it and throughout the whole experience I felt like Jo was all around me. It was the most wonderful thing and makes me cry with sadness and relief at the same time.

Anyhow, death is going to happen. I have a theory that actually most, if not all, of our actions are stemmed from our fear of dying. Our basic survival skills are there to allow us to stay alive; once these kick in then almost every one of our thoughts and actions is actually driven from a primal instinct to live. Fear in a relationship is actually fear of death – what do we do? We run for the hills. We fear someone at work, it triggers our sense of terror and safety; what do we do? We charge into conflict. Fear of death can subconsciously drive the decisions behind what car we drive, who we marry, who we don't marry, where we live.

When we get on top of those basic instincts, suddenly we can be really free to float through life. I say this as if it is the easiest thing to recognise and do. It totally isn't. It's kind of interesting to talk about for a few minutes, though!

Disassociation and Dissociative Disorders

We can all disassociate – or disconnect – to a degree. Think of the journey back home in the car. You finish work, jump in the car and you get home and realise you haven't really taken in the last twenty minutes of your journey because you went on autopilot and it feels a bit weird.

Disassociation can become more of a disorder when it persists for periods of time. For example, I got severe disassociation when I got PTSD and I couldn't recognise anything emotionally – I might know who someone was, but I would have no contextual feeling with it. It suddenly happened one day. I also couldn't recognise my face in the mirror; it was like looking at a stranger.

We dissociate for a number of reasons and essentially it is the body's way of protecting and preserving itself. During the journey home in the car, the body says to a bit of the brain, 'Don't worry, you can have a snooze – we got this.' If we are in a bomb blast, however, the body says, 'Let's leave our body immediately to prevent ourself feeling any pain.' Dissociation is our ultimate defence mechanism. Dr Livingstone, when he was being jumped at by a lion, described it as a 'painless dream'. When we are in a scary situation, something that is traumatic, we will often leave our body.

I write about this now as I believe these things are more common than people think. I had a disorder called depersonalisation. The symptoms of depersonalisation are not recognising one's reflection and not fully recognising friends and places, and it can lead to thinking and feeling that you are in a video game or some sort of film or that everyone else around you is in some sort of trance and only you can see what is going on. At its worst, it leads to major existential crisis and it can lead people to suicidal thoughts and depression and anxiety.

Derealisation is a less common dissociative disorder, where one's sense of bodily proportions is skewed and distances and objects change shapes and the way they look.

Dissociative disorders can be caused by trauma or emotional overwhelm. They can also be a reaction to drug taking, and this is especially common among younger men in their late teens to early twenties. Often people think they are 'going mad' and the disorders can lead to very internalised, complicated and damaging thinking. It is a very tricky disorder to get on top of, but just knowing about my own disassociation made me feel like I wasn't losing my mind. It is extremely difficult to get people to understand unless they have it, so to anyone who is or thinks they may be experiencing it, I would recommend reading a book by Dr Marlene Steinberg and Maxine Schnall called *The Stranger in the Mirror*, which provides a very comprehensive and in-depth examination of the subject.

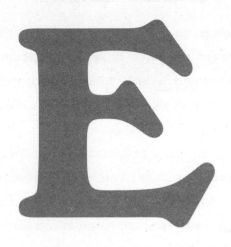

Emotional Hijacking

This is one of my favourite phrases and I have become fascinated with what can happen to move us into this state. Emotional hijacking occurs when our sensible, balanced mind is overtaken by a rush of past trauma. When something triggers us (see page 171), our brain gets flooded with old emotions of panic, anger, sadness or fear, and we stop functioning as an adult. We may experience a burst of rage or fit of crying that is not an appropriate level of reaction to the event that's occurred. (This is different to feelings of anger, grief or sadness that are an appropriate reaction to a real-life event.)

So, what causes an emotional hijack? It's all down to a reaction that takes place in our nervous system. I'm going to lay it out in basic terms because I'm not very scientific.

Our brain is made up of different areas: the back can hold a lot of trauma and is linked to our animal instincts of fight, flight and freeze, while the front brain deals with everyday stuff like motor function, language and problem-solving.

When we get triggered (and this can mean different things to different people), our brain will fire up, and old emotions stored up from the past will flood our system and can set off our defence responses. This is when the more survival-based parts of our brain that activate our caveman instincts can take over. Our rational thinking becomes obscured, so it is harder to be reasonable and in the present.

Here is an example of what emotional hijacking can look like:

Brian is going out with Steve. Steve has been hurt badly before in relationships and was cheated on. Along with this, Steve carries abandonment trauma from his childhood, which he has not addressed and which affects his behaviour. Steve gets very uneasy around Brian going anywhere without him and it has created problems in their relationship.

Brian needs to go on a business trip and although he keeps trying to discuss it with Steve, he finds he is being shut out and is unable to actually communicate healthily about what he is doing, where he is going and why and for how long. The trip happens and Steve says Brian is uncommunicative, selfish, just like all the other men he has been with, etc., etc. He then ignores Brian for the next month.

So, what has happened? Effectively, Steve's past unresolved feelings have come up to haunt him and his brain has fired up into a huge defensive response where he is not being rational, healthy or adult, and he has gone into a defensive shutdown. He is in full emotional hijack.

Our unresolved deep painful feelings can be so strong that they will flood our brain and our nervous system and lead to secondary defensive responses – responses that are possibly learnt behaviours that in the past kept us safe from the pain and reality of the original trauma.

So strong is the brain's defensive reaction that sometimes our adult brain – specifically the frontal lobe's ability to deal with the here and now – is taken 'offline'. This makes it genuinely difficult to be rational, remember details or clearly communicate and hear the other side of the story.

So, what can be done when you find yourself emotionally hijacked? The first step is to recognise that this can happen. Often this is aided by a therapist who can help you unpack what was actually going on, what you were feeling and what it might relate to in your past. Recognising emotional hijacking immediately helps us gain some mindfulness and distance.

Something I have experienced myself, however, is that as wonderful as having mindfulness is, it doesn't frigging stop the pain of being in a triggered, emotionally hijacked state. I would say when I was in treatment, 'Oh yeah, great, it's wonderful I know I'm in this state, but what the fuck do I do now?'

So, I write these things knowing it isn't as simple as it can sound. What knowing about the possibility of being emotionally hijacked *did* do for me was it stopped me acting like an arsehole! I didn't act on things when I was in that state, and that has been invaluable.

The next step is to work to bring down all that stored emotional pain, which means there is less and less to get triggered by.

But we will always end up getting triggered by stuff, so the key is to know what brings us out of it. For me, validation is a huge thing; sharing with someone how I am feeling (it's usually terror and hopelessness – such lovely existential emotions to feel!) and simply being heard brings down the emotional charge, often instantaneously.

We must also learn how to calm our system and bring ourselves back to present time. One way of doing this is by checking in with the senses. If any of these are uncomfortable for you or not possible, use the ones you can or find your own that are more suitable:

• Think about what you can smell and taste in this moment. I carry small testers of aftershave around with me because they very quickly get me back in the room.

- Sight-check the closest and furthest thing you can see. It can be as simple as looking around the room and noticing, 'there is my dining room table', 'there is my dog', etc.
- Touch objects around you and notice their different textures.
- Sound-check what you can hear nearest to you and furthest away.

Physically getting myself back into my body is also very helpful. I push my hands against each other or place my hands on the outside of my knees while pushing my knees against them to get strength into my legs.

Breathing is another tool we can use: breathe in for six seconds, hold for ten and breathe out for ten. Do this ten times.

Another idea is to go under a blanket. Often, covering our torso talks to our sense of safety as an infant. Or you can take a warm bath. Do some exercise. Drink water.

Discover what works for you and you will find you come out more and more quickly from emotional hijack. Sharing with your partner and friends what will trigger you into these states is also a great thing to do.

I do not underestimate how difficult it is because I experience it myself, and when two different parts of the brain are fighting with each other it's not easy. I do believe, however, that a lot of conflict within relationships and work and friendships and families comes from emotional hijacking. If people could at least recognise that it's something that happens to them, the world would be a lot more peaceful!

If you are involved in a situation where someone is emotionally hijacked, then I suggest first making sure you feel safe, and if someone is not being reasonable enough to hear you, then take a time-out.

Exercise

We all hear it and it isn't always as simple as 'Well, just go on a run, you will feel so much better.' It's not easy if you are down, and sometimes it can feel like you're dragging yourself through syrup just to get out of bed. Here is my little tip: you don't have to do exercise for a huge amount of time. There are programmes on YouTube called eight-minute abs, bums, arms, etc. You don't have to go full out; in fact, often this culture of pushing yourself to your limits isn't always that healthy. A small amount of exercise a day is great and can be just as good for you. It's the doing and the moving that is the key to getting your energy moving around. Twenty per cent of the oxygen created by exercise is used by our brain; it shows how important our brain is in function and what it needs to function well. Stretching is a great thing to do. Exercise can be anything: a light walk, or picking up bean cans and using them as weights! Take the stairs, not the lift. There are so many ways that you can exercise that'll work for you. Bugger what everyone else is doing, forget social media … you do you and notice what it does for you.

Expression

Expression is crucial. Years ago, when I was at university, I studied political theory. I wasn't the most diligent of students; however, I did enjoy reading various philosophers. I read Kant, Hegel, Aquinas, etc., and it was Karl Marx who made an impact with one of the simplest of things that seemed to really grip me. He wrote of the importance of putting something of yourself into your work, whatever that work might be. This I feel in part is to do with the importance of expression: we all need to express ourselves.

We need to express ourselves for several reasons. We have to get out what we have inside and this doesn't have to be only emotions and thoughts that are tough to feel. Think about it ... what do we do when we have some good news? We want to share it. We get a new job and we want to ring up a friend or family member or tell our partner, 'Guess what? I got the job!' This isn't about needing validation, it's about sharing with others.

It is harder when we have tougher emotions, which, if you think about it, is so silly really. This is something completely fabricated by Western society, in particular the notion that one should always be happy and the discomfort it gives to others when it is expressed that we aren't. We grow up being woefully ill-educated in identifying and expressing our feelings. Things thankfully have got better but it really should be something that is stringently placed on the school syllabus.

The reason I write of the lack of education is that we are in effect taught to ignore our tough emotions. What this creates is denial within ourselves and a splitting-off, so we react to ignore and invalidate our own painful feelings. This is why expression is so important because, if we don't express, we turn in on ourselves and this is where depression and anxiety come from; we collapse in on ourselves or move into a state of hypervigilance. It is essential to get our feelings OUT. Get the feelings out and keep on getting them out because, if left to swirl around inside, they will make us ill – emotionally, mentally, physically and spiritually. Speak your truth, draw your truth, dance your truth … however you express yourself, make sure you do.

The other important element to expression is to show the world who we are. To express ourselves is to show our authenticity. This is not always easy. If you are what is perceived as a minority and your very being represents your 'difference' to the norm, it is hard to become comfortable with expression. You must, though, and find your safe world where you can do this because by dulling our light, we again dull our spirit and our very being and become unwell.

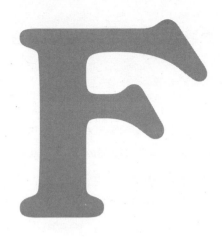

Failure

This is a word that I think should be banned. Perhaps they have now got rid of the letter F in the grade system at schools. I am not even sure what failure is apart from a way of describing an inability to succeed.

I either pass or I don't pass a driving test. I don't fail it.

I didn't *fail* at getting the job; I didn't get the job.

Failing denotes inadequacy and not being good enough at something. I see no purpose for the word to be used in any human context.

Yuck, get rid of it.

Family Systems

A family system is effectively made up of the different parts we play within our family. All families will have their varying characters simply by the mere fact we are all our own unique personalities.

A family system can become toxic or harmful when we are forced to take on roles to enable us to get by, to try to get the love that we need and crave as children. So, one becomes the perfectionist and the achiever, the well-behaved one. Another one might become the fixer, the peacekeeper, the problem-solver, and another can become the rebel, the 'failure', the non-achiever, the difficult one. Now some of these roles cross-pollinate but they mostly stay within their defined parts.

Ultimately, our role within a family system is a non-authentic form of self. To unpack this and see the character we have played to survive is an important step in the process of working out what we missed as children and discover who we truly are as adults. It's painful, yet ultimately liberating and fulfilling.

Fear

Here is another of the African Big Five.

Deep breath … and we are off.

Basically, I think a whole book could be written on fear alone. So I will say fear is, in my opinion, the biggest limiter in life and can be very simply broken down to a few areas:

1. Fear of rejection
2. Fear of failure (these are the two big ones)
3. Fear for one's physical safety
4. Fear that happens in the here and now
5. Fear that's been left in our bodies from past experiences and situations and our emotional reaction to those.

Fear is the bedrock of us as actual living animals. Our basic desire to thrive and survive is the most primal instinct, and fear is a necessary sensory experience to allow us to detect what is a threat and what isn't.

When our deep-rooted 'caveman' fear gets triggered – i.e. our body starts being told we are going to be eaten by a sabre-tooth tiger – different departments within our brain kick into gear.

When fear gets to a level that it overwhelms us, our frontal lobe – the management side of our brain – gets taken offline. This is when we can get lost; our thoughts may seem like a broken record and we can't seem to settle or find any conclusion to the perceived or actual problem. I call this the 'chain coming off the spokes'; we are pedalling yet getting nowhere and it is exhausting. Our nervous system gets heightened and we go into a fight-or-flight mode.

The problem when this happens is that we still try to think our way out of it. Our brain can't understand why we have gone into such a panic and, because it is a problem-solving organ, wants to find a solution. So, we think more and more, then we get more panicky, and it is an endless cycle.

So, how do we break this?

Well, we need to look at what can settle our nervous system. For me, these are the things that work:

1 I go right to the root of the problem and go to an acupuncturist or cranial osteopath, have a massage, maybe even do some light stretching and find release in doing some strength work to get back into my body and 'back in the room'.

2 Exercise really helps, especially if I am in full-on flight mode; a run can be just what my body needs!

3 I share my problems with someone who is actually going to hear me and validate what I am feeling.

Sometimes that is all I need – especially if I didn't get that when I was young.

It is very difficult to get out of the 'problem-solving' mode and look to calm our body, yet it is crucial, in my opinion, that we do that. The key is to settle our body by getting grounded, maybe by lying on the floor flat-out and sensing your back being supported, or lying on your back and elevating your legs onto a chair or up against a wall. Find some strength in your limbs by pushing against a wall, or try breathing in for five, holding for five and then breathing out for five. I imagine a square: I go up the left side breathing in for five, along the top while holding for five, then go down the right side while breathing out for five and along the bottom while pausing for five. (See page 106 for more on grounding.)

Some little things:

Fear of parties/social anxiety can often be about fear of rejection, i.e. 'people won't like me', or it could be a feeling that one isn't safe, in which case boundaries are crucial. (See page 34 for more on boundaries and page 150 for party nerves.)

Fear of failure is another big one – what happens if it doesn't work out? I might think, *People will judge me (and reject me)*. Then, I ask myself who worth knowing would actually judge and reject me for simply trying to do my best? No one that I want in my life – and if they have to be in my life I will choose to share as little of my time and thoughts as possible!

Of course lots of other things come into play. Fear of failure can lead to fear of losing money, fear of not being able to maintain a family, etc. Most of the time these things can be worked out and forecasting the worst-case scenario helps us to know what we are getting ourselves into.

As adults we are not allowed to feel that we can be scared. I certainly never, ever voiced or entertained that I could be scared. That was what children felt but not big, strong adults, yet of course we feel scared. Certain people can actually scare me and now I don't mind admitting it. I was too scared recently to embark on a conflict resolution face to face and actually stated this. I am completely within my rights to say to myself and others, 'I feel unsafe in this situation and I am taking myself away from it for my own wellbeing.' Anyone who doesn't respect that is not worth knowing.

Of course, we can't use this every time! I can't rock up to the counter at Starbucks and say, 'Sorry, I'm afraid I currently feel too scared to pay for this coffee and for my wellbeing, I will leave with my free coffee. Thank you.'

We have to be contained and listen to ourselves while always validating what we are feeling.

I feel scared about twenty times a day and I try as much as possible to validate it. Sometimes it is a younger part and that takes more time and energy for me to not reject it.

So we can have specific fears like fear of failure and rejection. We can have fear for our physical safety. We can have fear for our emotional safety and fear for something that is occurring in the here and now. And lastly, we can have fear that is trapped in our body from past events and may be triggered and overwhelm our nervous system. This is very nuanced and hard to catch but effectively it is post-traumatic stress, which you can read more about on page 156.

Learn to embrace the fact we feel fear, look to work out what it is you are afraid of and always validate yourself for it. If you feel scared then ... you feel scared, and it is for no one, not even ourselves, to try to take that away.

Feet

I know this may seem an odd thing to have in a well-being manual, yet I am telling you right now our feet are AMAZING things. If you think about it, when we walk or stand, we carry all our weight on our feet and so our body alignment comes from the ground up; our body shifts position dependent on how our feet are connected to the floor. This is why getting bare-foot at every opportunity is wonderful. Toddlers are the best example of being entirely connected to the floor. They spread their toes wide, almost frog-like, and this allows the feet to take all the weight of their body. As adults we press our poor feet into uncomfortable shoes, squishing our toes into heels and tight shoes so we can't find our balance, and it sets our body alignment out of whack. This in turn can affect our ability to breathe deeply.

I met a wonderful osteopath, David Warren, who taught me some incredibly simple exercises for my feet, which would help relax my body. You get a tennis ball and roll each of your feet on it, going up and down lengthways six times on each foot, making sure the tennis ball covers the whole of the foot. You then place the ball in the centre of your sole and go in a circular motion six times clockwise and six times anti-clockwise. Then repeat this on the other foot. Maintain a constant downward pressure as you do these three exercises and notice how your body releases and feels calmer.

A great way to calm yourself is to CALM YOUR FEET! Give yourself a warm foot bath and soak your feet for however long you want. Massage your soles with a simple oil or cream.

Another tip I have learnt, which honestly has helped not just me no end, but also two friends of mine who had huge difficulty sleeping … foot detox pads. I picked some up in a chemist because I thought I would try to offset my smoking habit by buying these silly pads. It said one of the effects can be improving sleep. I placed one on each sole – they are like teabags crossed with a plaster and, honestly, I slept so soundly and beautifully. In Eastern medicine, our feet hold a lot of importance and are given a lot of attention and I can understand why.

Look after the things that spend a lot of time under pressure – you won't regret it and your whole body will thank you for it. Allow yourself to 'take the weight off'.

Forgiveness

This is a big one – and I mean it really truly is a big one. I remember years ago beginning to knot all the pent-up anger and resentment, bitterness and jealousy that I had. I would hang on to things that had happened twenty years previously! I would hold on to resentments towards friends when it was actually my choice to do so. They didn't even know I was resentful!

Forgiveness is an act of movement, I believe. What I mean by that is that it is something that takes active participation. It might be through writing a letter and burning it, it might be by letting someone know how you feel, owning it and releasing that feeling of anger or hurt.

Many of us need to move through our hurt and pain to get to the stage of forgiveness. For some of us, forgiveness is key because otherwise feelings and pent-up energies can stay inside our body and that may tear us apart. I truly believe people can get ill because of pent-up emotion that needs to be resolved. I know I did. For others, however, the opposite is true. Forgiveness not only feels impossible but can be unnecessary or even counter-productive for their healing. In these cases, the person needs to deal with the emotions that have arisen from that event or action using other tools.

I have something currently that I am finding hard to forgive and I know it is because I never expressed my feelings at the time. I own that and it is my responsibility. I'm not sure I will ever feel safe enough to express this to the person and so I may write it down in a letter. It might have to take a few letters! I will get there, though. I will never send them, but I must get my anger out. Forgiveness, for some, is the most beautiful place to reach and it isn't always an instant thing.

Sometimes I tune into myself and ask myself, 'Can I forgive this or is this something I need to take to the next level and communicate it?' I am very good at communicating to others how I feel; however, I still get nervous about being rejected or being thought of as crazy or highly sensitive. I still have to remind myself that my feelings are valid, and through this I can reach a place of forgiveness where my body feels less weighed down. It is wonderful to feel light and unfettered. It isn't always easy and, my gosh, I have found that it is worth it. It is actually one of the greatest gifts we can give ourselves. Forgiveness isn't really about who or what we are forgiving; it is about reaching a conclusion and finding peace and closure.

Friendship

We hear it spoken of so many times – the importance of friendship. We are social animals, pack animals. It is good for us to connect with other humans. It is essential that we connect in a group and feel mutual love and appreciation and respect. This, to me, is what friendship is and should be.

Friendship is not having people who judge us or who lead us to feeling bad about ourselves or who just talk about themselves. Friendship is not having a friend who shames me all the time or doesn't show any interest in anything going on in my life, regardless of the emotional context.

Friendship is empathy. It is being able to sit with someone and just be. It is laughter and tears. If we haven't grown up with positive attachments, our learnt experiences of humans aren't necessarily positive. We sometimes need to learn that people can be trustworthy.

Sometimes, as we grow, we change and move apart from certain friends. This doesn't have to be a negative thing; some friendships simply run their natural course because lives go down different paths and there's no need to feel guilt or any regret about that. I have also chosen to end three friendships. None of these were done without careful thought and months of observing how I felt around them. Ultimately, I elected to actively end the friendships rather than simply ignore messages and become more and more evasive. That's what works for me. It is, I have to say, a sad and also liberating experience and feels fair to both parties concerned. Too often I think we live a lie and keep friendships while bitching about the person behind their back. If you feel you can't manage or don't want to do a conflict resolution, then lighten your load. Only with careful thought, I hasten to add! Otherwise it will be like kindergarten when kids are beginning and ending friendships every other hour!

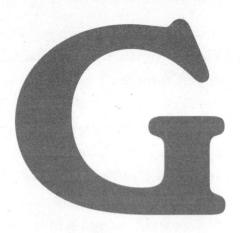

Garden of Life

(An odd one, but I feel an important lesson I've learnt and one I actually often forget.)

There was a monk who once wrote of the importance of keeping all the plants in your garden watered. The plants are a metaphor for different areas of our life. I have never forgotten this analogy and I like reminding myself of it: is one area of my life being over-watered and one under-watered? If I am feeling unfulfilled, I ask myself, 'How are the various areas of my life?' I like to think of my life as six categories: family; friends; work; spirituality; relationships; and my relationship with myself. Even as I write this now, I am noticing my spiritual side has been under-nourished of late and I haven't been good socially.

Something that comes to me when I think of these areas is: don't underestimate what it is like when one or more of them gets completely rocked. It so often can lead to us becoming completely off-kilter. Changing jobs or experiencing problems at work, losing a friend, having problems with a relationship, losing a parent. I often see it as if I am sitting on a stool: if one leg is slightly vulnerable then fine, but if it becomes two or three, that stool is crashing to the floor and I am going to be hurt! So often we can give ourselves a hard time, thinking we should be able to cope with everything, but we forget that we aren't infallible or invincible. We are, after all, human beings, not human robots.

So, keep an eye on your socialising; keep an eye on work and how much time and energy it is taking up; keep an eye on relationships and your desire to love and be loved; keep an eye on your family; and keep an eye on your connection to spirituality, whatever form that might come in for you.

Gardening

You don't have to be an expert to garden and – breaking news – you don't even need a garden! The beauty of gardening, or I should say growing, is it is ever evolving. It is magical and actually a sort of mini-representation of the miracle of life. If you have a windowsill you can have herbs or window boxes. You can plant bulbs in a little pot indoors; all you need is light and water. It gets you in touch with the rhythm of life, it slows you down and it is so fulfilling. To just touch some earth and enter into the simplicity of growth can do something for you. I'm not sure how, but when you get some seeds and then something comes to life from something so tiny, it can really work in just giving you a small task of mindful fruition.

Grounding

A word that is often bandied around is the importance of grounding. I'd never heard of it until about eight years ago. Grounding is about finding a practice that works for you that allows you to reconnect with the earth, get back into your body and then emotionally feel calm and grounded. It is a physical thing and an emotional thing. It really is a practice that could be done every day and often can be experienced through anything from stretching, talking with the right friend, cleaning, dog walking, lying on the floor … the list is sort of endless. It isn't that dissimilar to resourcing, yet what I would say is that it should have a particular quality of calm and almost a gentle heaviness.

Why do we need to ground? It allows us to re-centre ourselves and connect with the fact that we are OK. Often in times of stress we will leave our body and begin to float, and the more we become like a feather in the wind, the more easily things are able to blow us off-track. What I mean by this is that we can experience difficult emotions and so don't want to remain fully present in our bodies. The best martial artist will be completely grounded into the floor to allow themselves the opportunity to 'use' the floor when defending or attacking. Rooting oneself heavily into the floor literally means we are harder to push off-track. What it also means is that we have the ability to be lighter while coming from a place of deep connectedness, so everything comes from a place of peace and self-knowing. One thing I have noticed through all my training in performance, from voice training to dance training, is that the more grounded I am, the more I am able to be in control and therefore make the best choices.

The way that I usually find the easiest to ground is by lying on the floor and slowly letting my body feel gravity. I imagine the ground coming up to hold me rather than my body falling into the ground. I mean, obviously I can't do this at all times, but twenty minutes a day of doing this can be enough to maintain my centre.

Another relaxing exercise is to lie on your back with your bum up against the wall and your legs resting up the wall. Allow your lower back to gently caress the ground and feel a gentle blood flow to your upper body and head. It's a great thing I do in the dressing room when I have to wait around a lot before a performance; it helps keep my nerves calm.

When we encourage ourselves to be grounded, we find that everything we do comes from this centred place of self-assurance and peace and calm authority.

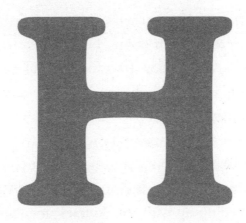

Home

I think a mixture of lockdown and Marie Kondo transformed how I approach my home. One of her benchmarks is to look at your possessions and see whether they invoke positivity and love; if they don't, chuck them. I did this with some surprising things; many of my awards, I realised, actually didn't hold any good memories or feelings for me, so I chucked them. The ones I kept mean so much to me, yet they are the smallest and seemingly least important of the bunch.

I talk to my home and I nurture it. I rub Danish oil on my furniture, and I give it a proper clean, skirting boards and all, at least once a year. I start every week making sure I brush off my front step. It's amazing what your home can become because it is your sanctuary and an externalisation of yourself. As I unpacked boxes six years ago in my present home, I said to my friend Tony, 'God, if this was a shop I would buy all these items', and his reply was, 'Well, that makes sense as you HAVE bought all these items!'

My home represents my taste, my travels, my finds, my loves. Take note about your house that you are doing it for YOU and not anyone else. It is so easy to get caught up in a 'keeping up with the Joneses' mentality, but so often I have been round people's houses and they are like show homes. There is no soul and everything there is to be shown off rather than enjoyed personally. There is a big difference between a house and a home; it takes time to make a home. A lot of this can be down to experiences you have in the house, but it doesn't mean you have to be a social animal; I certainly am not. I treat my house as one big mood board. It inspires me and comforts me. Make sure you feel supported in every room. You do you when it comes to your home as, after all, you are the one who has to live in it!

Hypervigilance

Hypervigilance is a term used in psychology to describe when we are in a state of heightened alert and become very sensitive to our surroundings. It makes us become aware of hidden dangers around us, such as from people or our environment, though often these may not be real. Hypervigilance can be seen as a symptom of extreme anxiety and is often linked to PTSD (post-traumatic stress disorder) and anxiety disorders.

Hypervigilance can also be known as hyperarousal. This is when the body is in a state of heightened awareness and 'jumpiness' and can lead to problems such as agoraphobia, insomnia, stomach issues, anxiety and depression.

Often, we can be running with a low level of hypervigilance and we might not even be fully aware of it. Other times, we might be in a full-blown state where any loud noise or person or even the presence of someone can be enough to set our nervous system into a full-blown panic.

It was fascinating to learn that a state of hypervigilance is easily related to a state of hypovigilance (see page 113) in that both are a reaction to something. Hypervigilance might be a reaction to a trigger – something that has come up inside me that causes my body to move into extreme anxiety – and then my defensive mechanism kicks in. A lot of the time I would be 'hyper', so in a state of fight or flight … I would feel a buzziness all throughout my body as adrenaline and cortisol got released. My appetite would be lost, I might get a runny tummy and need to go have a wee far more than usual. This is because when an animal is under attack, it doesn't think to stop and have a nice mouthful of grass while being chased by a cheetah! A reason that we will need to empty our bowels far more frequently stems, again, back to the animal kingdom, where it was essential to empty out the bowels in case we were pierced by a horn or tooth or claw and our body would become contaminated by our own waste. All I knew was that it gave me piles!

Hypovigilance

On the other end of the scale, hypovigilance (or hypo-arousal) is when the body goes into a protective shut-down mode. One feels lethargic, sleepy, but never 'nicely tired' in terms of feeling relaxed. One can experience what is termed as brain fog, where one can feel dazed and like the mind is surrounded by a sort of cloudiness.

Another reaction to something too painful and over-whelming is to go into a hypovigilant state – that is a state of freeze, fawn and collapse. It is, again, another response brought on by the body's ancient defensive mechanism. Often, when I was in this state, I would find myself developing brain fog, my body would shut down and I would become lethargic and depressed. It was never a 'nice' tiredness; more a sense of shutting down, like a computer.

Both hyper- and hypovigilance for me were, and still are, symbolic of my own reactions to overwhelming feelings based in my past that were left unprocessed. Learning to recognise these states was certainly a big help to me as at least I then understood what was actually going on.

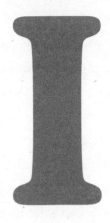

Instinct

People will speak of matters of the head and matters of the heart. Our instinct resides, however, in neither of these places; it is in our stomach. How often have you had a 'gut feeling' about something and it's turned out that that instinct was right? How often have you experienced a sense that you know something is or isn't right but you can't explain why?

When people speak about their 'gut instinct', there is some science behind it. Science has now shown that our gut acts like our 'second brain'. It contains millions of nerves and these nerves communicate with our brain and carry information up to it and back. In fact, our gut can influence our mood and our general wellbeing.

So, why is it so hard to listen to what our gut is telling us? The simple answer is we don't always want to hear it! However, once you tune into it and truly follow your instinct, you start gliding through life rather than swimming against the current. In fact, our instinct is extremely powerful and the more we tune into it, the more we can manifest and predict stuff. Sit right now and tune into it – tune into your stomach and notice it. What is extraordinary is our true instinct comes with NO JUDGEMENT and no affectation ... it just is. Our head will then jump in with perhaps predisposed emotional reactions, but our second brain just exists and guides in the purest sense.

The more we can learn to notice our head and work on past patterns, the more our instinct can rise to the helm and we can let go to simply let ourselves be guided through life.

Intention

Intention is everything. Honestly, it really is. Our intention for all that we do sets the agenda within us. We have to look within ourselves and be honest as to what our intention is for anything we do. What do we really want the outcome to be? But actually, perhaps more importantly, it is not so much about the outcome and more about how we want to get there.

I always say apologies are a great way to think of what our intention is. If I am apologising for something and I am doing it to fully own what I have done and that is all I want out of it, then it is a pure and healthy way of taking responsibility and seeing the benefits of owning up when I have done wrong. If I am apologising to expect an apology in return, or perhaps I am apologising to manipulate a situation, and I really don't believe I should be apologising, the intention is different.

Set an intention for everything. Ask yourself, 'What is my intention today?' and then look at it and think, *Is this the healthiest thing I want out of this?* Yesterday, I sang at a radio station's Christmas concert. As I travelled to the London Palladium I asked myself what my intention for the concert was. If I was looking to entertain people and the reason for this was to be liked and wanted and to feel worthwhile, then the purity of that day would have a different quality and perhaps not the most comfortable one. In that situation, I should challenge my intention – question whether it might be negative or manipulative and, if so, shift the intention to something positive, fulfilling and kind, both for me and the person who is the recipient of that intention. I decided my intention for the day was to help people. Years ago I saw a business coach, who allowed me to see that what I really wanted in life was to help people and that I could bring this intention to any line of work that I did.

On the surface singing could seem like something that isn't the most conducive to this, yet knowing my life intention and having this always underneath whatever I do brings me deep pleasure because with intention comes purpose. We all have a deep life purpose and when we work this out as our grounding intention, it carries over to everything we do.

Ask yourself what your intention is for whatever you are doing in a given moment, and use that exercise to see how kind, healthy, appropriate and loving you are being to yourself and the world around you. It is actually an incredibly simple yet eye-opening thing that has allowed me far more peace and happiness in my life.

Intimacy

Intimacy is not always easy. For me, the word 'intimacy' goes hand in hand with vulnerability. Intimacy isn't always what we think it is either. We can have sex and yet feel no intimacy whatsoever. We can be 'in love' and feel no intimacy. To be truly intimate we must be vulnerable – and, believe me, that's hard! To be vulnerable is to trust, and I have years of not trusting people close to me because of childhood experiences. We often mistake intimacy for other things – the rush of 'obsession' with someone or of constantly arguing with someone – because of what was modelled for us growing up. Check in with yourself, though; is this really what you want intimacy to be? Intimacy is feeling calm and trusting. It is the hug you want at the end of a day, the thoughtfulness of your partner and the support you provide each other. True intimacy is a wonderful adult state of mutual respect and support and advocacy. If we haven't experienced it before, it will take time to learn this, but my gosh, it is worth it.

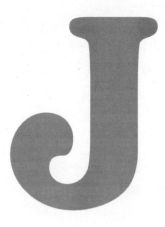

Joy

My friend says this lovely saying: follow your joy. I actually think I'm going to get it as a tattoo. It sort of simplifies life so beautifully and, really, life *is* that simple. What the saying does is allow us to have our benchmark and our rudder. Don't see it as much as a directive but more as an assessment tool. If you are feeling off at any stage, be it for a second or a whole year, ask yourself, 'Am I following my joy?' The answer might be 'I'm not sure what my joy is', and that is fine because it allows you space and an amazing opportunity to work out what your joy might be. For example, one of my decisions for this year was to finally go on a drystone walling course! I absolutely love drystone walls. I love the drystone medium as a texture used in art and also its functionality and its beauty. I love using my hands and I love the ancient tradition of the craft. It is my joy! So I am going to do it.

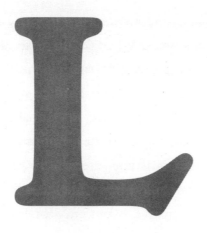

Love

I think Hollywood has a lot to answer for! It is not all *boom, pow* and there you are, magically in love with the person of your dreams. Now, of course it can be the case; I don't want to spoil your fantasies by saying it isn't always that way!

Often our sense of love is based on how we experienced love growing up. It took me a long time to realise that when I felt the POW moment and was convinced that this man was 'the one', I was actually just experiencing a huge amount of activation in my body. What I mean by activation is my anxiety and body memory of being emotionally abandoned was re-triggered by the person I saw in front of me.

We hold body memories in us all. They are not necessarily conscious unless we make them so, and so we can often misinterpret them. If my experience of love was to be abandoned, then when I am in front of someone who brings up the same sense, it can make me feel, more often than not, that the same thing will happen again. My nervous system is triggered into remembering that sense of uncertainty and anxiety. The difficulty is because this was my formative experience of love, of course I think that this is indeed TRUE love.

If I find myself on a date and I feel afterwards or even during that it is absolutely wonderful then it is certain that the person will not be the available one for me. It even happened the other day. My moorings became loose and I thought, *This could be the one!* My adult side kept an eye on it and I was correct that he was not interested in having another date despite saying he was. I say this with no anger … I let the old emotions take over.

To get used to a new kind of love I say is like turning the *Titanic*! For me, the less activated I feel after seeing someone (and the calmer I feel) tends to mean he is a better type of person for me. My body will tell me.

Often when we say I either fancy the wrong type of people or the ones that fancy me I don't find attractive, it is a sign that there is a need to change course. I am not saying I have the answer, because to date I have not! What I can say, though, is that I am much more content

NOT being in a relationship with someone who will abandon me emotionally, or indeed physically!

A few years ago, I was in the beginning stages of a relationship and we were staying at a hotel together. While my new partner was in the plunge pool that came with the room, I said from the shallow end of the pool that I was feeling quite anxious that day. After sharing this I watched my boyfriend move backwards away from me until he was up against the far end. I chuckled to myself because I thought if there was ever a sign that he didn't want to be or wasn't capable of being present for my emotional state, here was a clear one! We broke up a week later. Incidentally he did it with an emoji via text, which was new to me!

So the basics of love are ... fizz and sparkle are absolutely fine when you meet someone. If you find relationships more a pleasure than a chore, you don't argue constantly and are emotionally present for each other, then enjoy that spark! If you find you are unable to maintain relationships or find them difficult and triggering, then be observant of those moments when there is deep intensity from the off. Listen to your body and tune in to how you are really feeling about what your desires are. Feeling constantly anxious and nervous and intense is not always the best kind of love and can be detrimental to your wellbeing.

Physical love is a good thing to look at as well. I had a relationship once that was incredible in the bedroom department, yet we argued constantly. I was never actually fully present for the sex; the fire came from the energy of constant abandonment between us.

Notice what you perceive and feel love to be. We all get blueprints from our childhood/prior experiences and sometimes they don't aid us in our future endeavours for love. Love can look very different to different people, even within the boundaries of healthy frameworks. Look at your own blueprints, but also don't feel your experience of love has to fit in with what society presumes it will be like.

Love Addiction/Avoidance

When people think of love addiction they often move quickly to sex addiction. This is largely because they have probably never heard of it, so I think this is a very important entry not only to clear up what love addiction actually is but also to show how I think a lot of people might relate to it.

Put very simply, love addiction is just that: 'addiction to love' – a reliance on the individual's personal notion of what love is and what it can do for them. The typical pattern of a love addict is to instantly feel a rush when they first meet someone and feel like they have met 'the one'. They will often say after just one date, 'You know, I really feel this is it.' They experience a bubble of love, obsessing about the person and feeling a rush or high, and believe that everything has suddenly come into focus. The reaction that love gives them is literally like that of a drug. The chemical and emotional reaction is heightened and also short-lived. For this is the next stage of love addiction.

Certain patterns of thinking and behaviour will emerge after the initial connection. These could be anything from constant ruminations on the other person to thoughts of worry that the person will leave – or alternatively, that the person is getting too clingy. A love addict can start to compare themselves unfavourably to their love interest, they might start getting possessive, or they might start going completely the other way and become distant and avoidant. The love addict can go from being deeply invested to disinterested in the blink of an eye.

Some people might think, *Well, this is just the usual behaviour or falling in love,* and yes, sometimes we do fall into a rush of endorphins and feel intense emotions for the object of our desire. The trick, however, is to look out for patterns of behaviour. For example, if someone says to me, 'Well, we've met and we are moving in now after three dates and I really think this is the one', I don't judge; however, ninety-nine times out of one hundred I will start to see the warning signs of love addiction and the bedrock of an unhealthy relationship beginning to form.

Where does love addiction come from? I think a lot of it is based on attachment patterns and intrinsic wounds of abandonment from childhood, where the person is still looking to resolve what was never met emotionally. The problem with this is that often we are attracted to the same type of person with the same emotional responses as our original caregiver who hurt us, and so the pattern continues.

There is some fantastic literature out there for sex and love addiction and even twelve-step groups like SLAA (Sex and Love Addicts Anonymous). Pia Mellody speaks and writes very eloquently and knowledgeably about love addiction. My rule as someone who was a love addict and still has that propensity within me is to notice that 'rushed' feeling when I meet someone as it's something that most likely is not healthy for me. If I am feeling instantly on a high, then it is possible the person is not the right one for me.

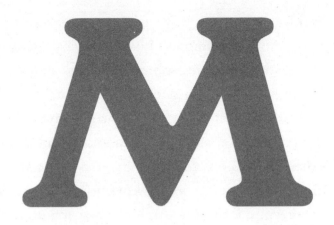

Martial Arts

I think practising martial arts is an amazing way of getting to feel one's sense of boundaries. We get into our balance and our sense of being grounded. We learn to breathe, to feel the ground, we learn respect. When I started Muay Thai kickboxing, it was not because I wanted to kick people's heads in or to discover some hidden power within myself; it was to get fit. I went out to Thailand with my brother to spend time together in a different way by exercising in the morning and sitting in the sun and exploring in the afternoon. What was fascinating to me was that I came back from the camp three weeks later feeling a palpable shift in my self-confidence out on the streets. For me, as a gay man, I had experienced my fair share of homophobia and it was often scary. A skill like this will, of course, never prevent anyone being the victim of abuse, and although I have never had to use any of the skills I have learnt, something in me shifted. Just knowing I have them has given me more confidence.

A misconception about martial arts, perhaps, is that it's aggressive and about looking to attack, but this isn't my experience. The key is to never go seeking any sort of fight. It focuses on training, repetition and remaining calm and centred, because this is the best way to remain at one's best in case one does ever get attacked. These teachings are then carried into life, outside of training. It really is rather remarkable. We see this in very calm activities like qigong and tai chi, which were designed to be used by fighters and employ similar power moves.

Money

Money is the root of all evil is what they say. It's not fully true but it can make things very tricky for a number of reasons. Especially if it is hard to come by. Rich people sitting there saying, 'Oh, money isn't everything', are very irritating. Money is needed and makes life a hell of a lot easier if you have a lot. It is seductive, money, so what I would say is watch out if you start earning more; when this happens, your life grows so you have to spend more, and suddenly your expenses are massive. Before you know it, you have to earn more money to simply exist and so the capitalism trap is set. Happy people don't spend money, or certainly not on unnecessary things. Just because we earn it doesn't mean we have to get the bigger house or faster car. Keep an eye on your relationship with money. There is no shame in wanting a lot of it; just make sure you're using it for the right reasons.

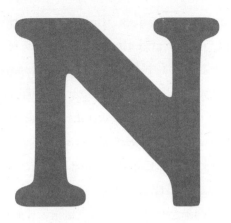

Needs

Recently, I have been fascinated with the notion of neediness. I openly have needs. They range from food, shelter and water to the essential desire for connection with others. These are different connotations to neediness. As an adult, if someone is 'needy', they have an unbridled and uncontained desperateness. This spills over into a lack of boundaries, heightened emotional responses and immature behaviour.

Children are needy in a similar way. I certainly was. I constantly craved attention, physical affection and validation that I was loved and cared for. Often this would spill into what could be called 'showing off', and sometimes it was rejected, or my desire for love and validation was not met with the appropriate responses.

Neediness in an adult that is overpowering, just as in a child, is one and the same thing. It relates to a key phrase: UNMET NEEDS. Put very simply: unmet needs are when a child does not get resolution to what is needed. Most of the time, I would wager that what the child is looking for is a feeling of safety and security. If a child isn't receiving the love and attention it needs, it means it isn't safe. With this kind of survival drive running underneath an unmet need, the desire for resolution is never-ending. It will stay, I believe, in the body until it is recognised and defused and understood and continually shown it has a new route to resolution that doesn't need to include fear, panic and terror.

In my opinion, an old UNMET NEED is a soul wound, a desperation that has such energetic ferocity that it can ruin our adult lives without us even knowing.

The issue with UNMET NEEDS is that they can become an injured part of us that is split off from ourselves ... by ourselves. To get on with living, we have to bury the pain and the terror and all the feelings that go along with the abandonment. For an unmet need IS abandonment. Once a part of our emotional history and experience has been split off, we have to work very hard to get through many defensive layers and find the original pain. This is what my brother calls the Hero's Journey.

We must wrestle with our minds. Our brains are set to be problem solvers. It has taken me five years to see that when I feel an overwhelming neediness, the enhanced emotion is from the past and therefore nothing to do with what is actually going on in the present. The brain wants to disagree and this is something that can be attained by practising mindfulness – getting more and more used to observing your thoughts and feelings. This is how for so many years I was trapped in internal conversations about whether a person was right, or whether he was wrong … should I date this man or that man? etc. It would drive me crazy. Underneath it was actually a constant triggered unmet need looking for resolution and never being able to find it.

Learning that it was OK to be needy has been an amazing lesson for me. I still feel a lot of shame about it. I often feel I should be able to completely rely on myself and no one else. However, I see more and more the power of connecting with others, owning my neediness from the past and present and finding healing through that. What we want to do is work to heal unmet needs from the past and validate our needs in the present.

Neighbours

Relationships with neighbours can be complicated. It's great to have wonderful neighbours, but often we are forced to live alongside people we just don't get along with. The key to keeping things smooth in these situations is to avoid passive aggression at all costs. I remember a neighbour I once had who couldn't just say something outright. They smelled smoke in their house and they thought I was smoking in my bedroom and it was coming through to theirs. I said to them, firstly, I wasn't and, secondly, I would be within my rights to smoke in my bedroom if I wanted to. They were dreadful at actually saying what they wanted to say, so any issue was always pussyfooted around. I made it very clear to them, if you have a problem please just bring it up as I can only react to that. They were key at passive aggression.

Once, I had my parcels left at their house and they sort of grumbled about it but weren't really saying anything outright, so I asked directly, 'Would you like to not accept my parcels because I am absolutely fine with that – could you just clarify this so I can organise myself accordingly?' I have NO time for passive aggression or lack of clarity, so my rule is to look for clarity and then I will act on the information I am given. If my neighbour wants to hate me from within their house and yet present differently on their front step, I have no problem with that as I will act with the information I am given. We don't have to have these huge confrontations; we can approach things in a mature manner and also allow others to have their feelings.

But don't sit there and get more and more annoyed at your neighbours and not say anything to their faces because you will simply make yourself ill and they won't even know what is wrong! Of course, if your neighbours are really inappropriate, aggressive, violent, etc., then authorities must be brought in. And ultimately, if you really are having your life destroyed by a neighbour, then move if you can; life is too short and you will be so much happier.

Nervous System

This is my sort of geeky fascination. I'm obsessed with my nervous system. Largely because eight years ago it started going berserk! The nervous system is our body's main communication centre. It controls our movement and thoughts, as well as some of the body's other systems and processes, such as breathing, blinking and digestion. It's basically a network of nerves that receives information from the world around us, then it processes that information and triggers reactions, such as making our muscles move or causing us to feel pain.

What I've also realised is that my nervous system is fundamental in how calm I am feeling. It's our nervous system that prepares the body for fight, flight or freeze, and it's a different part of the nervous system that restores the body to a calm and composed state and prevents it from overworking.

Most of my days are spent making sure my nervous system knows that all is OK in the world, be it through exercise, grounding techniques, voice work, drawing – anything where I'm expressing myself.

Sometimes it is harder than other times, yet I have realised that as important as my brain is, my body and nervous system are just as important. Ask a GOOD therapist what comes first, the thoughts or the nervous system being activated, and you could be there for some time! Whatever the answer is – and I think the answer is: it depends – don't forget the importance of your nervous system. Think of the phrases 'nervous breakdown', 'frayed nerves' … if we are all jittery then it is very hard to feel content, peaceful and happy.

Let your body do the talking and see what it needs. So often, just resting my back on the ground for ten minutes can reset my nervous system and I know that all is OK, not through my mind but through my body calming down. People say eleven seconds of hugging is enough to calm our nervous system. We are fight-or-flight animals and so, just like horses or gazelles, we need to remain calm. Often our nerves go off on one when they don't need to, so we need to show our bodies it's OK. Massage your feet, your neck. Honestly, by treating the body, I have often found the mind actually takes care of itself.

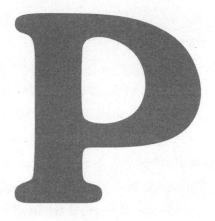

Parents

I think the most useful thing someone ever told me was 'Don't expect from people what they are not willing or capable of giving', and this is an amazing thing to remember when around parents. In some way or another, our parents most likely will have affected us in a less than healthy way – it is the way of human nature. Even the most well-balanced, stable parents with good attachment styles and emotional awareness will affect us and annoy us on occasion – and often even trigger us.

One reason for this is that we can get caught in the trap of looking for the thing we never got growing up, and by doing this can enter a sort of subconscious stand-off with our parent or parents – an energetic fight where we are still seeking that elusive thing, be it praise from our father or the words 'I love you and am proud of you' from our mother.

I actually wasn't going to put a section about parents into this book, and then a friend came to me recently to talk about his family. So, I thought I would describe what he went through – keeping my friend anonymous, of course – and then look at what was going on and how one could navigate this situation. It's complicated because not only did the situation involve the usual family dynamics, but it also occurred at Christmas, which can be a very charged time for families (see more about Christmas on page 45).

Here is what happened: the day before my friend was due to go home, his father rang and was in a hugely triggered state. He hadn't slept with worry due to something and went into attack mode towards his son. He was shouting, shaming and attacking. The next day, the son went home and was promptly greeted with monosyllabic answers from his father and whispered vicious insults from his brother, who also would deliberately block him in the kitchen. He observed how his mother and brother would converse with each other in whispers (a common practice of theirs); they would then make overly polite conversation with my friend, but it would be peppered with eye rolls whenever he would say something in return.

Eventually my friend left two days after Christmas, and when we spoke he asked me if I thought he had made a mistake in not addressing the failings and painful words and behaviour of his parents over the years, stuff that had come up for him through therapy. I sat and thought about it and then asked my friend what his intentions would be in addressing those failings. It was clear his goal was to try to receive some recognition from his parents of where they had not been great in bringing him up and how they had hurt him. I asked him if he thought they were capable of that, and the answer was no.

Often, when people go into rehab, they will have a family week where relatives – most likely the parents – come and have a dialogue that is overseen by a neutral party in a safe capacity. Both parties can feel heard, and hopefully, some stuff will shift. If we don't have this, it is often extremely difficult to give the kind of feedback my friend wanted to give without falling quickly into old patterns and reactions. If this is something that one feels needs addressing, then I strongly urge people to use a third party as it allows for a safe space where neither party feels attacked and both feel heard.

Even so, sometimes we will never receive that missing piece we seek from a parent – be it affirmation, an apology or some sort of explanation for past behaviour. When we make peace with this, while being empathetic to our younger parts that never received that recognition, we can truly forgive our parents, and this is when your relationship can reach a better place. (Although, it should be said that sometimes parents can do unforgiveable things. If you are in recovery from any kind of abusive treatment in your childhood, for instance, forgiveness isn't the only option when coming to terms with how your parents have affected you.)

For my part, I didn't realise how much anger towards my parents I was holding inside myself until I went on an eight-day experiential course, and my gosh, I released a lot! After that my relationship with my parents, which was good but loaded with pent-up anger from being sent to boarding school, went from strength to strength. I'm not saying it's perfect, but I go into interactions with them protected against the potential things that might upset me and allow myself to receive the great stuff as well as give it.

For example, if the need arose, I might set a boundary with my father by saying, 'I would rather you didn't speak to me like that.' If my intention with this was to state my truth with love, then I will have done just that. I might go further and say what I would do if I were spoken to like that again, and that is still a very clear and clean statement and practice. If, on the other hand, I said those words but expected a wild change in behaviour in return, or deep sorrow on my father's part for sending me to boarding school, I would not be being pure in my intentions and would most likely be setting myself up for a fall. (It's actually a common thing we do in all areas of life. We say one thing, yet really what we are wanting is something else; and then when we don't get that something else, we resent the people for it, even though we never made it clear in the first place!)

So, when it comes to dealing with parents, remember this: keep your side of the street clean; come with love, not with anger; and don't expect from others what they are not willing or capable of giving.

Parents-in-Law

One word … boundaries! You have to remember that your in-laws are your partner's actually lawful parents whether they or you like it or not! It is not easy and really the key is for everyone to stick to their lane. It's a great American saying, which my friend uses. You get on with your job and they get on with theirs. The bottom line is no one should have to put up with any rudeness and inappropriate behaviour, and to do this you must set boundaries with love; you can't lose your shit because once you have then you have no right at all to expect others to keep their shit together.

If it gets to a stage where you simply cannot be around your in-laws, then there is no reason why you should have to be. Let them see the kids but as much as possible keep yourself safe and away from toxicity. The key to the whole thing is actually to be united and mutually supportive in your relationship; parents are triggering but you must let your partner calmly know and hear how you feel and what the repercussions can be. Try not to get into using your partner to tell your in-laws stuff that you could be telling them; when it comes to boundaries and emotions, this doesn't work that well and keeps conflict bubbling away under the surface. Also, try and find common ground – look for the love and try being forgiving. Give yourself support and time limits if you have to be around in-laws you can't bear so you don't feel trapped; things can be easier when you know there is a treat at the end of it.

Party Nerves

I give myself ten minutes at a party. I know that for the first ten minutes I will be uncomfortable. When I was badly socially phobic, I employed a great CBT technique, which was to score out of ten how bad I thought the party experience would be and then score it when I returned from the party. Along with this I would score how anxious I was feeling before the party and how anxious I felt afterwards. What this did was it allowed my mind to see that feelings do change, that they would always lessen in strength and that, actually, emotions like joy and fun would creep in.

I do have a rule, however, that if I am feeling particularly anxious, I won't stay at the party. I also tell myself, 'You don't have to go.' Often just hearing that I don't have to go calms that scared part of me down and suddenly I feel more like going! Often we just need to hear that we aren't being forced to do anything. When we know we aren't in a hopeless place and do actually have control, our anxiety diminishes.

Positive Attachment

Years ago I had my first experience of positive attachment with a partner. He was American and his emotional intelligence and way of communicating were extremely impressive. He normalised having mature adult dialogue around his inner and outer world, and for the first time I felt like I was forming a positive attachment with a partner.

Positive attachment for me is feeling a sense of continuity, regularity, support and safety with someone. It is having someone who validates and hears you, allows you to have your emotions, doesn't look to fix and is capable of standing next to you and witnessing you in all your true emotional form. It is being with someone who has healthy boundaries, who is able to have difficult conversations without going on the attack or the defensive, and primarily who makes you feel seen and heard.

If this was something that wasn't modelled for you growing up then you can find these positive attachments through friends, maybe a great boss, through a religious or spiritual figure if you are religious and often through therapy and hopefully with a partner. It might take you a while to get used to being with someone with a positive attachment style; the key is to be curious about how you feel after being with someone. Do you feel calm or heightened, anxious or content or depressed? Notice every time and read *Attached* by Dr Amir Levine and

Rachel S. F. Heller, then you can start doing your own mini quizzes and assessments of other people's potential attachment styles – with love and kindness, of course.

Processing

'Processing' is a term for working through and finding a new conclusion or approach to old emotional wounds and trauma. We need to process stuff that has happened to us not only by using our mind but also by allowing the body to work through past traumatic energy, as the muscles and nerves hold on to memories just as much as our brain does. This can be done in a plethora of ways: talking therapy, journaling, EMDR (eye movement desensitisation and reprocessing), somatic work, body work, acupuncture, cranial osteopathy, group therapy. Experimental courses such as Survivors, the Hoffman process or exposure therapy … the list is really endless.

The key with processing is to know that it CANNOT be rushed. Be very wary of any promises of being fixed in six weeks. This is especially true when working with past traumas; there are still too many theorists who promise instant results through exposure therapy, and in my opinion this is a very dangerous thing. When we are exposing ourselves to past difficulties and possibly deep emotional pain that we have subconsciously buried for years, it can be extremely overwhelming, so we need to work with someone who is safe and gentle and will not push or rush us.

Projected Emotions

I learnt about projected emotions a long time ago and it was a bit of a game changer for me. At the time I was going out with someone and they would spend a lot of time calling me selfish. I could, of course, be selfish at times and I was not the perfect boyfriend. Later on in life, however, I would hear from people that they actually found this person selfish. This is, by the way, not throwing him under the bus because I write this with love and it is a good example for me to use.

So, what are projected emotions? Effectively, when someone doesn't have full awareness of their emotional state and patterns of behaviour, they will project what *they* are actually being or doing onto the other person.

A basic example – a friend steals my photo frame and in response will accuse me of being a thief.

Another example can be the partner that will berate their other half for never listening and yet the reality is it is they who is unable to be present and listen. Projected emotions can often come up when people are anxious. My friend would get very anxious when walking around a town on holiday, and often she and her husband would get into an argument over this. However, the argument would have nothing to do with the topic of her being anxious but something different entirely. The original anxiety was never dealt with or owned by her. This is a different type of projection when the person does not have control of their emotional state and so will lash out at others. It is caused by uncontained emotions and ends with the anxious person on those closest to them.

Projected emotions can become extremely dangerous in relationships and can lead to what is called gaslighting, where one person is effectively berating and brainwashing the other person to such an extent that the victim believes they are actually what they are being called – be it self-ish, uncommunicative, etc. This can happen because the partner being projected at wants to love the 'projector' so much that they lose their own identity and sense of self. They essentially get bullied. It isn't necessarily someone who is weak-willed who gets gaslit; they might be highly functional in life and at work, but in relationships, such is their desire to make it work, they lose themselves to keep the peace, or they find themselves trapped by an abuser or their circumstances.

To stand firm against emotional projection, we must remember we are enough with or without a relationship. Otherwise, co-dependence will creep in and allow us to become needy to the point of toxicity. We have to work on our own boundaries and maintain our own space so that other people's actions will remain on their half of the street.

PTSD

PTSD (post-traumatic stress disorder) is a much larger topic than perhaps people first think. It is, in a nutshell, past traumas catching up to the modern day, hence the term 'post-traumatic stress disorder'. Symptoms include a shutting down emotionally to a numbed state, loss of interest in things that used to excite and interest you, less of a desire to be around people, visual and emotional flashbacks, loss of appetite, trouble getting to sleep or trouble waking up, bowel problems, intense headaches.

PTSD was initially recognised not only in response to the Vietnam War but also around the same time by prominent feminist writers who spoke of latent trauma in relation to domestic abuse, and so PTSD was even at its birth related to more than just war veterans. Trauma, as defined by Jo Stubley – a consultant psychiatrist in psychotherapy and head of the Tavistock Trauma Service (part of the NHS Tavistock and Portman Trust) – can not only leave you feeling hopeless and helpless and in existential terror and pain but also make you lose your trust in people and the world. One of the great things she says about trauma treatment is you don't ask what is wrong with the person; you ask what happened to that person. Therefore, treatment for PTSD takes on a whole different therapeutic approach.

Treatment for PTSD can sometimes involve medication, to help with the problems of anxiety or depression, as well as talking therapy, CBT that is specially designed for PTSD, EMDR, somatic therapy and group therapy. Some people have even used psychotic drugs like ketamine and MDMA, and indeed, some have said that shamanic rituals like ayahuasca ceremonies can have huge benefits. However, these things should NOT be taken lightly – especially if the person is on any medication – and should be heavily researched to ensure the person is being looked after.

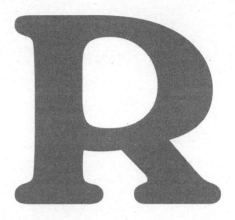

Resources

Resources are things that we have in our life that aid us in remaining grounded. For example, today I am in my attic studio writing this as I can get hypervigilant and so being in my little 'den' feels safe. Who knew that my attic would become a resource for me?!

It's a bit of a 'therapy speak' word, yet I find resourcing useful to remember because it reminds me there are things I can do to help myself. My list of resources is like my tool belt. Some days the resource I need might be talking to friends, other days it could be having a hot bath or stroking the dog. Be curious about what is resourceful for yourself and build up your list.

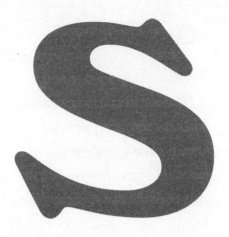

Sage

White sage being burnt is a wonderful clearer of a space. After I was burgled I burnt sage throughout the house. If anything traumatic happens, or even someone has been in your space who has bad energy, burn some sage. Energy stays in the corners of the rooms, so make sure you get the sage smell in the corners and clap in each corner to remove the bad vibes. Sounds bonkers but it works, I promise!

Self-Esteem

There was a great talk I heard by the guru who is Pia Mellody. She's written on love addiction and co-dependency and I remember her saying something that really stuck with me. When it comes to self-esteem you are either in it or you are not; you are either experiencing self-esteem at any given moment or you aren't. It isn't something that operates on a sliding scale. Different to confidence, self-esteem, she said, cannot be labelled a 2 out of 10 or an 8 out of 10, and this really stuck with me. It stuck with me because, similarly to asking oneself in the Buddhist tradition, 'Am I living in fear or living in love at this moment?' it causes me to ask myself, 'Do I have self-esteem at this present moment or do I not?' It forces me, in a way, to get to the root of a problem very quickly. Often, I struggled with the notion of being present because, frankly, it's difficult! Especially when in an emotional hijack (see page 79) because when my nervous system is flooded with activation, I find it extremely hard to bring myself back into the room without the aid of someone else. What I have always liked, however, is this simple act of being present and asking myself, 'Where is my self-esteem at right now – is it present or lacking?' Ask yourself this question when in any situation because often just this simple act can ground you.

Settling

A 'settling' of oneself is a term I like to use. To feel settled is to feel calm, physically and mentally. It's like coming home to how the body can be. For me, I like to think of settling as my nervous system reaching a place of a good flow of yin and yang, where my chakras are open and working together. Essentially it means a calmness has descended over me. People talk about settling down or finding a place and that is where they decided to 'settle', but, actually, it is such a lovely word to apply to our emotional state too.

Shaman

Shamans are also known as witch doctors or healers, depending on where they practise or their origin and where they learnt their craft. Shamans largely come from South America and look to use animal metaphors to relate to human power and movement. They work closely with nature and believe in the power of the planet and use of the wider natural world to help guide, support, heal and strengthen. A wonderful book by the shaman Jo Bowlby, called *A Book for Life,* gives a great, simple introduction to shamanic thinking.

Shamans use sounds and smells a lot in their practice to help bring the body back to a peaceful state, as well as soul retrieval to heal old wounds and even trauma passed down through the generations. Many people are uncertain and possibly even scared of shamans, but I have found, with my shaman, the practice to be anything but scary – not even that weird, just wholly liberating and relaxing.

Some people go on to practise ayahuasca ceremonies with a shaman, using plant-based medicine to have a psychedelic experience that is set to open the consciousness and even reset the nervous system from past traumas. I haven't done it personally and would recommend you take extreme precaution and that you go with the right person. A ceremony should NOT be in a huge group and you should have at least one shaman present to guide and support you through the ceremony, which can last for hours and hours.

Somatic Therapy

This is a therapy that has saved my life, I would say. When I first came across it, it quickly made sense to me. People can think that it is more hocus pocus than science, yet it is truly a scientific reality and very much grounded in biology.

Somatic therapy looks at the connection between the mind and body and uses physical therapies to bring about holistic healing. Along with talking, somatic therapists use mind-body exercises and other physical techniques, such as dance, yoga, meditation and deep breathing, to help release the tension that is negatively affecting one's physical and emotional wellbeing. Somatic therapy can help people who suffer from stress, anxiety, depression, grief, addiction, problems with relationships or sexual dysfunction, as well as issues related to trauma and abuse.

The idea behind somatic therapy is that our nervous systems, and therefore our bodies, can hold on to past traumatic energies. Unlike in the animal kingdom, where traumatic events are quickly dissipated from the body, unfortunately for us humans, our big old brains get in the way, often preventing us from allowing the completion of an energetic cycle.

For example, take abandonment; an abandoning experience in childhood will lead to a flooding of adrenaline and cortisol into the body. Until we feel safe again, this energetic surge will continue to flood our systems. In somatic therapy, by bypassing the mind and going straight to the body, we get in touch with this initial feeling. With the support of a therapist, we allow the energy to dissipate and also allow our feelings of helplessness to change, finding a new conclusion. In effect, we can rewrite our own history through this amazing experiential therapy.

Through this treatment I rewrote my history at my detested boarding school. It took two years and I was taken back to the time I was there; all sorts of feelings and visions would come up. Slowly I managed to leave the classroom, then get to the car park, then finally to the end of the long school drive where the outside world awaited me and, with open arms, all my present-day friends were cheering me on! It was amazing!

What somatic therapy does is get us out of our heads. Our problem-fixing brain is an amazing tool, however, what often happens, is that it can take us in the wrong direction. For example, mine would sense the alarm bells ringing from my nervous system and think, *Right, I have to fix this. Clearly something is wrong*, so I would then move house, buy a new car, think I needed a new partner, and so on. By getting to what I like to call the 'dandelion root' of the issue, we stop this endless reverberation of fight or flight, fawn or faint or freeze and find a new conclusion.

It truly is magic. It ain't easy, though! It is something we just aren't capable of doing by ourselves. We need someone to be there with us, allowing us to test the water.

Try it if you are able!

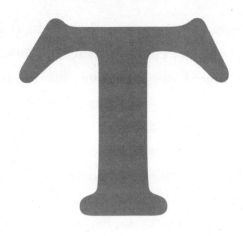

Trauma

Trauma and its definition have come on a long way over the last ten to twenty years. Essentially, trauma is the experience of something that leaves us feeling helpless and hopeless. We can have big traumas, such as natural catastrophes, accidents, war, physical attack, etc., which can be a one-off event, like a hurricane, or a sustained, repeated event, like ongoing physical or sexual abuse. We can also experience little traumas that are not seen as such a big deal on paper, yet the overriding emotion is one of being powerless and helpless and hopeless.

What I have learnt is that it is not for anyone to define what anyone else's trauma is. If I found dropping some eggs in a supermarket traumatic to the point of feeling existential helplessness, then that is what I feel. Too often we get caught up in the story and actually ignore the emotions. These are emotions that are often stuck and need processing. Trauma is trauma, the feelings are the feelings, and we are all allowed to experience our feelings and have them validated.

Childhood trauma is often something that can set in and have an enormous impact on our wellbeing; indeed, many believe trauma to be at the basis of 99.9 per cent of addictions. Childhood trauma can be caused by abandonment, or a lack of healthy constant attachment with one's caregiver/s, and it can create huge developmental problems, which come out in later life in depression, anxiety or behavioural problems such as addiction.

'Trauma' is a word that has, because of its sense of grandeur, led to many belittling the idea that they might have experienced it. Take the grandeur away and focus on the difficult feelings underneath. Once we can process these, we can free ourselves up to live clearer lives. For more on how to heal past trauma, see page 153 on Processing, and page 166 on Somatic Therapy.

Triggers

Here is the thing about triggers: a trigger is something that might happen that creates a response in our mind and in our nervous system that can be more powerful dependent on how old the stuff is and how much we have worked through it, as well as how severe the trauma was and how severe the triggering event is.

For example, I went out with someone who was Belgian. Now, if someone gives me Belgian chocolates (this has actually happened), I get triggered in my mind by the association. Because I worked through my grief over the ending of the relationship, the trigger is minimal; the association comes up in my mind, but the ensuing emotional pain at this thought is one per cent of discomfort – because I took the time to properly grieve.

Here's another example. Autumn is a season that is very triggering for me. It actually is classic textbook PTSD, where memories buried deep in my mind, memories I buried out of survival, begin to resurface. My body is overwhelmed very quickly by a flood of adrenaline, hopelessness, fear and high anxiety. Occasionally I may get a visual flashback as well as emotional ones. Me sitting in the classroom, me being in the car park, looking at the driveway, willing myself to run away but knowing I can't as I will just be brought back and punished. It is murky and messy and I begin to feel suicidal. I know this is a symptom.

This is an example of being triggered to a much deeper state of pain and terror, one which is over thirty years old, and I am still working on processing it through proper trauma therapy. I need to reach out to my therapist or a friend to explain what I am feeling, try and make some sense of it, connect to it and find myself back in the real world, as in the present day.

Every trigger and its ensuing state should be validated. What we must not do, though, is get to a stage where we use our own personal triggers as a way of controlling others. We can set boundaries; however, we can't use our stuff to try to manipulate the world around us and almost use it as a weapon or a raison d'être. It is a fine line.

When I was in treatment, there would sometimes be things that would come up on television that would trigger someone in the house. We worked as a group, with the aid of a therapist, and would listen if someone perhaps was triggered by a food programme, due to their history with food, or perhaps a model competition, due to their history with self-image.

We would discuss how best to move on from this. Sometimes we would agree to change the channel and other times we would reach an agreement where we would let certain housemates know when a certain triggering show would come on, thus allowing them the time and space to move somewhere else for an hour. We wouldn't binge-watch the series but just watch one hour's worth and then they could return. If I was triggered and demanded that the WHOLE house never watch food programmes – or in my case, it was reality talent competitions (at that time, by the way, it was triggering, and I feel I must say talent competitions were NOT the root of my traumas!) – it would be unreasonable, demanding that the tail wag the dog.

My point is we will all be triggered at some stage; I will be triggered every day. I can't change the season autumn, I can't change being around certain people, but I can change my behaviour. We must be mindful of our triggers.

Another little tip: usually the bigger the emotion, and the harder it is to pinpoint to something in real time, the higher the likelihood I'm being triggered by something from my past. If I'm feeling something very strongly, nine times out of ten it will be an old unresolved feeling that has surfaced and created emotional hijacking (see page 79).

Twenty-Four-Hour Rule

This is something I am NOT very good at! It actually can be used for a number of things. I can be quite reactive sometimes, although I have got a lot better. In fact, to be honest, sometimes I think I react because it acts as a distraction from another uncomfortable feeling state I am in.

Now, I often try to enact the twenty-four-hour rule when I am asked to make a decision at work: I ask how immediate the need for an answer is and if it isn't something that needs urgent attention I will ask for twenty-four hours to think on it. It gives me space.

The other times this is useful is when I receive either an email, message or some news that angers and upsets me. When this happens, I try not to immediately act on it but give myself twenty-four hours. I must say I do find it difficult, and I guess the hardest thing about it is actually living with my anger and upset feelings. I have to remind myself to never act on anger in my mind or heart because it invariably ends in a fight!

There is, however, a more serious and, I guess, useful lesson to all this, which is that I use the time to allow myself to contemplate and then tackle whatever is needing my attention from an appropriate adult position. What setting twenty-four hours does is it can act as an external boundary and it also acts as an internal boundary to myself and my little parts that want to have a good old slanging match. It is actually something that is invaluable to me and something I learnt from my dad; we have more time than we think and we are allowed to ask for it. He would often say to me, 'Just give me a minute on that as I actually don't have an opinion on that.' It's a great phrase to use, especially if we are in a meeting or a conversation and we are losing our way or things are spiralling. We are allowed to take time in all aspects of our life, and if others want to rush us, well, let that be on them.

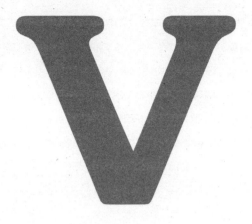

Validation

Validation is the recognition and acceptance that another person's (or our own) thoughts, feelings, and behaviours are understandable.

This is one of my elixirs of life. When we have feelings and we do not feel heard or validated, it can trigger a wash of shame and send us into a vortex of worse feelings. There is nothing worse, in my opinion, than having feelings invalidated and this is at the core of so, so many conflicts. Check in how many times people actually do or don't validate your emotions. I have a friend who I share with and that person will reply, 'Oh, that's a shame', and actually I am not looking for them to put an emotional response onto my emotions but just to be heard and for my feelings to be acknowledged, rather than dismissed.

Check in with how many times you actually feel heard and validated. It won't be as many as you think. Feeling validated is different to being RIGHT. Validation is neutral; it means that your emotions matter, your emotional state matters and therefore shows that YOU matter. It is something we as humans are simply dreadful at, yet it is so important.

Voice

Our voice is ESSENTIAL to us. Think of what we use our voice for: self-expression. Finding my voice was something that was life-changing for me. I saw voice coaches for acting jobs and realised I wasn't really using my voice to its full extent. Follow voice exercises on YouTube and notice the different colours in your voice; we have SO many. We use our voice in so many extraordinary ways. I lower my voice when correcting my dogs; I remain calm, yet I ensure they know I am being stern. We never need to shout in anger. Shouting means a loss of control. Get control of your voice and you will start to realise you can use it for so many things.

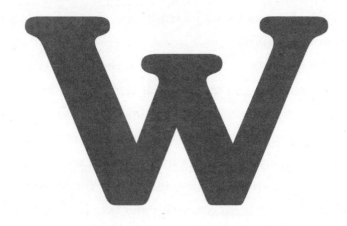

Work

It's so easy to say, when it comes to our working lives, 'Oh, just find what you love doing and all will be fine. Don't think about the money, think about your happiness.' Yes, how lovely to be able to do that; HOWEVER, we all have families, mortgages, debt, things we want to do, etc.

We all know money doesn't equal ultimate happiness (though I will say it makes life a hell of a lot easier). However, I for one am fed up with wealthy people – or people who are extremely privileged, running lifestyle businesses when they also have about fifty nannies for one child – telling others to just do what they love and not think about money. They can get lost!

Still, we have to face the fact that we spend a large portion of our lives at work, so it's important to be mindful of a few key points to increase our chances of feeling happy and fulfilled.

The first I would say is that you should try your best at what you do – no matter what that is – while remembering that your job does not define you.

One of the only things I remember from studying Marx was that he talked about the importance of putting something of yourself into your work. When I was a pot wash boy as a student, I actually did take pride in being a pot wash boy. If I was going to do a job, I was going to do it the best that I could. Don't let your sense of what a job means for the 'type of person you are' get in the way of taking pride in your work. Your job does not define you. Be the best at what you do and try your hardest.

So, ideally, we want to be putting something of ourselves into our work, but if you can't and you're doing a job just for the money, make sure you are getting fulfilment elsewhere. If you're working to put your kids through university, make sure you get the actual time to see them. Make sure you spend quality time with people and that you have fulfilment outside of that job. Obviously if your job is making you ill, then this is a different thing and you must leave work if you can; however, when we find we are working in an unfulfilling job and are also bereft in other areas of life, this is when we become destitute.

Work can be our passion and our vocation, or it can simply be a pay cheque that enables us to do other things. Check in with yourself and see if what your work is enabling you to do is actually making you happy and satisfied. Also, check in as to why you are doing the job you do. Are you trying to impress others? We are NOT our work title. There is a friend of mine who introduces every friend with their job title and it always pricks my curiosity. It is nice to know what people do in their lives, but I don't live in a world of top trumps where I think I should pay more attention and respect to someone based on what they do for a living!

I noticed after a few years of being a pop star and actor that I was basing a lot of my happiness and my sense of identity and self-worth on the job that I did and the money I earned. Then, at some point, I clearly remember thinking, *If this goes and I suddenly can't fly first class or go to posh places, what would I be left with and how would I feel about myself?* This is when I started therapy! Now, the idea of wrapping my self-worth in my earning capacity and work feels so precarious. I still sometimes let my ego get in the way and think, *What are other people thinking of me? Shouldn't I be driving a posher car and living in a bigger house?* The truth is, when I was living in bigger houses, yes, they were lovely, but I was miserable! I cared so much about how people saw me that I couldn't actually enjoy my work. It was a lose-lose situation. Now, I take every day as a blessing. I am grateful, and that gratitude staves off my insecurity about not being good enough, not being as successful as I was, not selling more records and not being more famous. Gratitude allows me to be in the present and think, *Wow, I can't believe I get to do this job!*

Another work lesson I stand by is not to lose your moral compass and subscribe to the old phrase 'nice guys finish last' because, to be honest, nice people – even if this were true and they did finish last – tend to be a lot happier and fulfilled and like themselves a lot more.

Twenty years ago, my friend joined *Vogue*. I remember ringing her at work on the landline and when she answered her manner was so offhand and bored: 'Hello, *Vogue* ...' Who knew just two words could give connotations of 'Hello, why the fuck are you calling me? My time is precious, I'm better than you – *we* are better than you – what the HELL do you want?'

I said to her, 'Are you aware you're answering the phone like this?' She said that was how everyone there answered the phone, and I replied, 'Just because everyone else is being an arsehole doesn't mean you have to be!'

I use this as an example of how often in work we are set examples of behaviour and language that would never be tolerated in the outside world. I have been guilty of it. I thought I could be a certain way and speak a certain way because that was what one did at work. I thought feelings didn't come into it. Yes, in many ways feelings don't have to come into work because business is business and often feelings can muddy the water. But it is never appropriate to belittle others or abuse one's power.

I wish I could come up with practical solutions for how to deal with difficult bosses or employers/employees (I do talk a little bit about bosses on page 32), but, really, it's not my area of expertise. I don't experience this world as I work for myself mostly. What I can say, though, is communication is key in all aspects of life. Try to resist the passive-aggressive emailing (like the classic 'As I said in my last email ...'). Ask yourself every time if you really need to be bothered with the aggro of something or if you can let it go. There are times when, yes, you need to put your foot down. It is, however, never acceptable to lose your temper, and work so often condones this. How well you treat people should not be dependent on whether you are in a boardroom, or your home, or a restaurant. You can still be firm and treat people with kindness. Shaming people publicly or privately is not acceptable.

Another thing I learnt recently is the complication of mixing friendship and work. It is not impossible to do, but often the way people communicate at work is very different to how they communicate outside of work. This is separate from whether someone is rude or not. The kinds of questions, for example, a boss might ask are very different to those a friend would ask. I would never ask a friend how many hours they had done that week and if they had filled in their time sheet, yet as a boss I am completely within my right to do so without it creating a problem. But when we try to integrate that boss-employee relationship into our friendships is when lines can become blurred. Be mindful of what you communicate – and also when – but the old adage 'Don't mix business with pleasure' can so often ring true for a reason. Sometimes combining the two simply doesn't work.

One final note: so often we forget how far we have come in our careers and what wisdom we have gleaned along the way. A really good thing to do is to look into mentoring others and passing on the lessons you have learnt in your work and life. Helping others on their career path allows you to see how much knowledge you possess and to actually find deeper value in yourself and what you do. I would highly recommend it.

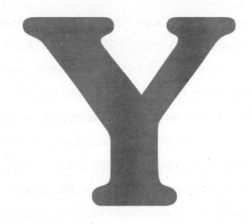

You Make Me Feel

I do not at all want to spoil the illusion or indeed the beauty of the Carole King song '(You Make Me Feel Like) A Natural Woman' and if anyone hasn't watched Aretha Franklin's final performance of that to honour Carole King, please stop reading and go find it on YouTube. Do come back, though, because this one is an important one.

Years ago, I remember my brother coming back from rehab and saying to me, 'You know, no one can actually MAKE you feel anything.'

I didn't get the concept until I started getting better at making boundaries and noticing my own co-dependence. To take the song in question, there is a huge difference between stating 'When I am around you

I feel like a natural woman' and 'You MAKE me feel like a natural woman'.

The key thing is ownership of one's emotions. In fact, the semantics of being made to feel isn't really the key issue; the issue is that by recognising that I have emotions that are mine and mine alone, the response in my body and my subsequent actions are also mine and mine alone. I need to be clear that there are, of course, situations in which our feelings *can* be manipulated – in the situations described above I am not including any forms of abusive behaviour and the effect it can have on a person's feelings.

Here is another example: someone opens their car door into mine, denting and chipping the paint of my brand-new Ferrari. I step out and feel disappointed and angry because this car is my dream car and I have just purchased it that day. I worked twenty years to get the car of my dreams and someone who is on the phone and not even paying attention slams their car door open. The person is not sorry in the slightest and in fact turns round and says, 'Fuck you' to me as I ask for details. I fly into a rage and to prevent the person leaving I rugby tackle him to the ground, pull his hair and give him a Chinese burn. I then take my keys and scrape the word 'ARSEHOLE' in his car door and end up getting arrested. At the end of the day I say to the police, 'It isn't my fault, he made me angry.' An extreme example and, I stress, not a real one. My reaction to the man's actions is mine alone. The disappointment was mine, the anger was mine, flying into a rage was mine and the rugby tackle, Chinese burn and key vandalism were mine. This man did NOT make me angry or MAKE me do any of those things. The man DID make a dent in my car door and chip the paint. The man DID show complete disregard for his actions and he DID act inappropriately, childishly, aggressively and shamefully.

Let's take the same actions: same thing happens and the only difference is I have just stepped out of an hour-long massage. I'm feeling relaxed, calm, grounded and have perspective on what is important in life. My door is dented, the man is aggressive and I feel sad, frustrated, a bit scared and wary, and I choose to simply let him go, ask for witnesses, take the details of his car and go on my way to report it to the police and ring up my insurers when I get home. The man did NOT make me relaxed or grounded or sad, frustrated and scared. The massage enabled me to feel relaxed and grounded, and the man's actions brought up feelings of sadness, etc.

I might have even observed that I felt sorrow and pity and love for the man. My point is our emotions change constantly, and when we see that the stuff that is coming up inside us is not FORCED by someone else, we get greater control and responsibility and overall mastery. It then shows us that we also have mastery of our actions.

I was interviewed by a researcher the other day for a TV show. Often before going on a TV show they will have a person call you up to do a pre-interview so the presenters have information and, if I want, will provide a list of questions that will be asked. I actually don't really care about knowing the questions and often the whole thing is rather dull. Often it will be a type of person ringing up who really has little to no interest in what I have done for the last twenty years; they literally couldn't give a shit. On this occasion, the woman was junior, rude and dismissive and it really, really upset me. I felt invalidated, worthless, pointless and really didn't want to go on the show, to the point I was sick and having a major panic attack on the day of the show. After unpacking it with my therapist, I realised I was hugely triggered into a past state of feeling uncool and completely useless. The person had not made me feel any of these things; if I hadn't been so tired or whatever I may have brushed it off, but in that particular moment I reacted emotionally. Was the researcher rude? Yes. Was she dismissive? Yes. Could she give a shit? No. My feelings, though, were mine and mine alone. By owning our feelings we reclaim the power because, let's remember, often when growing up and continuing into adulthood people try to manipulate and control our feelings. Parents or bosses or work colleagues might try to shame us, scare us, or intimidate us to garner power.

This one is CRUCIAL to actually realising you have self-mastery. It is not for someone else to control your emotions and actions. By recognising that no one makes me feel anything, I can realise that I am in the driver's seat. I can be kinder to myself. I don't assign blame onto others. I take responsibility for my shit and I keep my side of the street clean and I validate my emotions. I won't let others invalidate mine, and if they do ... well, it's not always pretty and that's something I need to work on!

Own your emotional world, own how you react and know that no one can MAKE you feel anything and then suddenly there is a whole shift to your self-empowerment. It is actually rather wonderful.

List of Resources

Books

A Book for Life: 10 steps to spiritual wisdom, a clear mind and lasting happiness by Jo Bowlby

Attached: Are you Anxious, Avoidant or Secure? How the science of adult attachment can help you find – and keep – love by Dr Amir Levine and Rachel S. F. Heller

Breakup Bootcamp: How to transform heartbreak into healing by Amy Chan

Breath: The new science of a lost art by James Nestor

Facing Codependence: What it is, where it comes from, how it sabotages our lives by Pia Mellody

Feel the Fear and Do It Anyway by Susan Jeffers

Healing the Shame That Binds You by John Bradshaw

Stranger in the Mirror: Dissociation – the hidden epidemic by Dr Marlene Steinberg and Maxine Schnall

The Body Keeps the Score: Mind, brain and body in the transformation of trauma by Bessel van der Kolk

The Feeling Good Handbook by David D. Burns, MD

Websites

Bacp.co.uk
The British Association for Counselling and Psychother-apy; a really useful resource to find an accredited coun-sellor or therapist.

Mind.org
A charity providing advice and support to anyone experienc-ing a mental health problem. It also campaigns to improve services, raise awareness and promote understanding.

ptsduk.org
A charity in the UK dedicated to raising awareness of post-traumatic stress disorder – regardless of what trauma caused it.

Relate.org
Relationship support for people of all ages, backgrounds, sexual orientations and gender identities, helping them to strengthen their relationships.

Youngminds.org.uk
A UK charity fighting to ensure children and young people get support for their mental health when they need it.

Helplines

National Suicide Prevention Helpline UK
0800 689 5652

Samaritans
116 123

SANEline
If you're experiencing a mental health problem or supporting someone else 0300 304 7000

Switchboard
If you identify as gay, lesbian, bisexual or transgender
0300 330 0630

Index

3 5 7 9 10 8 6 4

Ebury Spotlight, an imprint of Ebury Publishing
20 Vauxhall Bridge Road
London SW1V 2SA

Ebury Spotlight is part of the Penguin Random House group of companies
whose addresses can be found at global.penguinrandomhouse.com

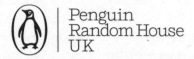

First published by Ebury Spotlight in 2022

www.penguin.co.uk

A CIP catalogue record for this book is available from the British Library

ISBN 9781529148374

Printed and bound in Great Britain by Clays Ltd, Elcograf S.p.A.
Imported into the EEA by Penguin Random House Ireland,
Morrison Chambers, 32 Nassau Street, Dublin D02 YH68.

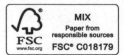

MIX
Paper from
responsible sources
FSC
www.fsc.org
FSC® C018179

Penguin Random House is committed to a
sustainable future for our business, our readers
and our planet. This book is made from Forest
Stewardship Council® certified paper.